SUPPORTING SELF C
PRIMARY CARI

Ruth Chambers
Gill Wakley
and
Alison Blenkinsopp

With the Working in Partnership Programme

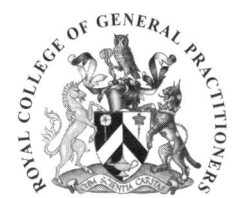 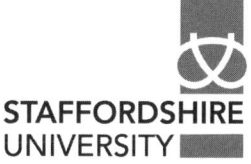

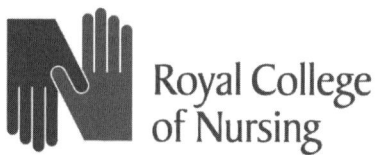

Foreword by
David Colin-Thomé

RADCLIFFE PUBLISHING
Oxford • Seattle

Radcliffe Publishing Ltd
18 Marcham Road
Abingdon
Oxon OX14 1AA
United Kingdom

www.radcliffe-oxford.com
Electronic catalogue and worldwide online ordering facility.

© 2006 Crown copyright, with the exception of the material listed on p.iii, which remains the copyright of Ruth Chambers and Gill Wakley.

All rights reserved. No part of this publication may be reproduced, stored in a retrieval system or transmitted, in any form or by any means, electronic, mechanical, photocopying, recording or otherwise without the prior permission of the copyright owner.

Ruth Chambers, Gill Wakley and Alison Blenkinsopp have asserted their rights under the Copyright, Designs and Patents Act, 1998, to be identified as Authors of this Work.

Neither the publisher nor the authors accept liability for any injury or damage arising from this publication.

British Library Cataloguing in Publication Data

A catalogue record for this book is available from the British Library.

ISBN-10 1 84619 070 3
ISBN-13 978 1 84619 070 4

Typeset by Advance Typesetting Ltd, Oxford
Printed and bound by TJ International Ltd, Padstow, Cornwall

The material listed below remains the copyright of Ruth Chambers and Gill Wakley.

- Chapter 3. Entire section on 'devising an education and training framework for the PCT in relation to the promotion of self care', including Figure 3.2 and Boxes 3.3, 3.4, 3.5 (pp. 35–41).
- Chapter 4. Section on 'building your team', including Box 4.2 (pp. 47–9).
- Chapter 5:
  Section on 'developing and sustaining an effective communication style', including Box 5.1 and Figure 5.2 (pp. 54–6).
  Section on 'sharing decision making', including Box 5.11 (pp. 60–4).
  Section on 'helping people change', including Figure 5.3 (p. 65).
  Section on 'demonstrating your competence in relation to self care through a personal portfolio', including Figure 5.4, Box 5.14 and Box 5.15 (pp. 69–72).
  Section on 'matching your knowledge and skills to the Agenda for Change framework', including Box 5.16 (p. 72).
  Section on 'illustrative example of evidence to demonstrate that you are competent at enabling patients to adopt self care' (pp. 72–4).
  Section on 'communicating risk to patients in relation to self care', including Box 5.17 (pp. 74–6).
  Section on 'time management' (pp. 76–7).
  Section on 'self care for you too ...' (pp. 77–8).
- Chapter 8 in its entirety, including all tables (pp. 114–17).
- Chapter 9 text in its entirety, including all tables (pp. 118–22).
- Tools 1, 2, 3, 4, 5, 6, 7, 8, 9, 10, 11, 12, 14, 15, 16, 17, 18, 19, 20 (pp.173–228 inclusive, excluding Tool 13).
- Appendix 2 in its entirety (pp. 236–38).

Contents

Foreword	vi
Preface	vii
About the authors	viii
Acknowledgements	x
About the Working in Partnership Programme (WiPP)	xi
Abbreviations	xiii

Part 1	**Making self care happen**		**1**
Chapter 1	Supporting self care *Ruth Chambers*		3
Chapter 2	What we know about the practice and impact of self care *Ruth Chambers*		14
Chapter 3	Getting organised for supporting self care as a primary care organisation *Ruth Chambers*		30
Chapter 4	Getting organised for supporting self care as a general practice team *Ruth Chambers*		43
Chapter 5	Getting organised for supporting self care as an individual professional in the general practice team *Ruth Chambers*		53
Chapter 6	Getting organised for promoting and supporting self care as a pharmacy team *Alison Blenkinsopp*		81
Chapter 7	Seeing self care from the patient's perspective *Ruth Chambers, Health First and Matthew Critchlow*		101
Chapter 8	Managing change – moving to a self care culture *Ruth Chambers and Gill Wakley*		114
Chapter 9	Completing the cycle: evaluation *Ruth Chambers*		118
Part 2	**Illustrative patient pathways to self care**		**123**
Chapter 10	Illustrative patient pathway to self care: sore throat *Gill Wakley*		125
Chapter 11	Illustrative patient pathway to self care: back pain *Gill Wakley*		136
Chapter 12	Illustrative patient pathway to self care: asthma *Gill Wakley*		146

Contents

Chapter 13	Illustrative patient pathway to self care: cough and colds *Gill Wakley*	159
Part 3	**Tools to help you plan and support self care** *Ruth Chambers and Gill Wakley*	**171**
Tool 1	Force-field analysis	173
Tool 2	Devising your PCT/practice strategy and action plan to establish a new culture of promoting and supporting self care	176
Tool 3	Strengths, weaknesses, opportunities and threats (SWOT) analysis	181
Tool 4	The basic planning process: taking account of political, economic, sociological and technological (PEST) factors	183
Tool 5	The gap model	186
Tool 6	Plan, do, study, act (PDSA) model for improvement	188
Tool 7	Timetable tasks with a Gantt chart	191
Tool 8	Infrastructure and resource matrix	194
Tool 9	Undertake an audit of how well established support for self care is in your practice	197
Tool 10	Training needs analysis	200
Tool 11	How well is your team functioning?	202
Tool 12	Significant event audit	204
Tool 13	PART/workload assessment	206
Tool 14	Moving through change	211
Tool 15	Keep a reflective learning log	213
Tool 16	Reduce time pressures at work	215
Tool 17	Check out whether self care support is a priority for training and whether the way in which you plan to learn about it is appropriate	217
Tool 18	Draw up a personal map of support mechanisms in your life	221
Tool 19	Assess your consultation skills and style	223
Tool 20	Determine your consulting style	226
Tool 21	Self care aware consultation style: encouraging, guiding and providing support to patients to adopt self care	229
Appendix 1	Useful resources	234
Appendix 2	Record sheet to plan and describe your progress in supporting self care	236
Index		239

Foreword

Many of our patients would benefit from, and indeed welcome, more information and support for self care – advice on lifestyle changes, how to manage minor ailments or to better self manage their long-term medical conditions.

There is evidence to support claims that more confidence in dealing with these challenges will improve quality of life for such individuals, but also it can give them better self esteem which, in itself, leads to better health. If you agree and/or you wish to explore what self care entails and how best to support it within your practice, this book is essential reading.

It sets out a training programme for general practice and pharmacy teams as a route to a practice culture where promoting and supporting self care is integral to every aspect of the healthcare and services the team provide. As a result of this programme, the team will be aware of the evidence for supporting self care, knowing what works and what is worth trying. It will also be well coordinated so that everyone is giving out similar advice and thinking of all aspects of a person's health. This might be by preventing a condition arising in the first place, by helping them manage their condition themselves as far as they are able, with treatments they can buy over the counter or initiate themselves, or by living with the symptoms until they improve spontaneously or tolerating them as part of every day life.

The training programme is a great resource for any primary care organisation or practice, GP, nurse, pharmacist or other health professional who wants to champion the support of self care. Its success relies on a good strategy and action plan, with enough enthusiasm across your team for the time and effort it will take initially. In order to get you started, the book provides four worked examples of how to help and support patients to self care if they have asthma, back pain, cough and colds or a sore throat.

Reading this could literally change your (working) life. Evidence shows that once support for self care is in place and your patients are taking more control of their healthcare, you should notice the drop in demand for unnecessary consultations, but, more importantly, this book can improve your patients' health and wellbeing.

I strongly recommend it and congratulate the authors on such an excellent contribution to enhancing primary care.

Dr David Colin-Thomé
National Clinical Director of Primary Care
June 2006

Preface

About the training programme to enable primary health care professionals to support self care

This book is a guide for anyone involved in commissioning or providing primary care, to help them understand what people can do to care for themselves or those they look after. Then they can set up systems in the primary care organisation (PCO) or their practice to support self care and enable patients and the public as a whole to self care whenever possible.

Self care is about people's attitudes and lifestyle, as well as what they can do to take care of themselves when they have a health problem. Supporting self care is about increasing people's confidence and self esteem, enabling them to take decisions about the sensible care of their health, and avoiding triggering health problems. Although many people are already practising self care to some extent, there is a great deal more that they can do.

The key is having health and social care professionals enthusiastically supporting self care. A practice needs all the team to be signed up to advocating self care and finding ways for patients with all kinds of health conditions to be able to self care. This book explains the importance of self care and its potential benefits in managing demands on health services by patients. It guides you to undertake self care effectively as a PCO, as a general practice or a community pharmacy team, as a practitioner, seeing the patient's perspective, learning to manage change and evaluating your progress and achievements. There are 21 tools to help you establish the self care culture that you will need, and four illustrations of patient pathways to self care – on sore throat, back pain, asthma and cough and colds.

The book is a part of the multidisciplinary training programme for health professionals to learn to promote self care, and introduce self care support interventions for common health conditions in their patients. The book is an additional resource to the online training programme for general practice teams and PCOs. You can look online (www.wipp.nhs.uk) to see how to run working groups or action learning sets for your colleagues – all the materials you will need are there. Download the facilitator's handbook from the site if you have lead responsibility for establishing and learning about self care, especially if your practice or PCO aspires to establishing a self care culture and not just a one-off try at self care.

Go on – try it.

Ruth Chambers
June 2006

About the authors

Ruth Chambers has been a GP for more than 20 years and is currently Director of Postgraduate General Practice Education for the West Midlands Deanery, and Professor of Primary Care at Staffordshire University. The focus of Ruth's academic career has been to develop education and learning initiatives for the NHS that fit health professionals for practice. She is the education lead for the NHS Alliance. Ruth has undertaken research and written widely on ways to encourage patients to be involved in managing their own health and wellbeing; and to contribute to the development of NHS services. She led the Staffordshire University team who were commissioned by the Department of Health Working in Partnership Programme to evolve this training programme for health professionals and managers on supporting self care by patients.

Gill Wakley started in general practice in 1966, but transferred to community medicine shortly afterwards and then into public health. A desire for increased contact with patients caused a move back into general practice, together with community gynaecology. Throughout she has been heavily involved in learning and teaching, adding some academic primary care later in her career, becoming a visiting professor at Staffordshire University. Like Ruth, she has run all types of educational initiatives and activities from individual mentoring and instruction, to small-group work, plenary lectures, distance learning programmes, workshops, and courses for a wide range of health professionals and lay people.

Alison Blenkinsopp has researched and written widely on self care since qualifying as a pharmacist in 1981. She has research interests in extended roles for community pharmacists and patient experience of pharmacy services. She led on the evaluation of patient experience in the national community pharmacy medicines management study. Alison's work on self care includes several reports, and along with Ayesha Dost she developed a compendium of examples of self care support for the Department of Health. She is one of the academic advisers to the Department of Health Working in Partnership Programme and a member of the steering group for the Joining Up Self Care project.

Alison is Professor of the Practice of Pharmacy at Keele University, a post she has held since 1999. Prior to her work at Keele she was founder Director of the NHS Centre for Pharmacy Postgraduate Education for England.

Matthew Critchlow and *Health First*. Matthew has a PhD in animal biology and has worked in the health care sector (both NHS and industry) for the past 16 years. More recently, Matthew has worked as an independent consultant in the health promotion field, as well as being co-ordinator and trainer for the Expert Patients Programme.

About the authors

Health First is a specialist NHS health promotion agency serving Lambeth, Southwark and Lewisham and hosted by Lewisham PCT. Health First works in partnership with health and social care providers, local authorities, and voluntary and community organisations to improve the health of local populations and reduce health inequalities. The agency offers advice and consultancy, opportunities for learning and development, access to a specialist health promotion/public health learning centre as well as a variety of other services linked to health promotion.

Acknowledgements

We gratefully acknowledge the help and input from colleagues in the five primary care trusts (PCTs) that piloted the self care skills training programme for health professionals – North Bradford and Airedale PCTs, Lambeth and Southwark PCTs and Central Cheshire PCT. We thank members of the Working in Partnership Programme self care steering group and project management for their guidance and feedback including: Clayre La Trobe, Helena Stone, Drs Pete Smith and John Chisholm, Ayesha Dost, Gopa Mitra, Louise Jarvis, and Lynn Joels from Medicom. Especial thanks go to Sara Buckley, the Staffordshire University project manager, who contributed to the production of the training programme with support from university colleague, Barbara Brown. Thanks to Christine Glover, Robert Hallworth, Alastair Buxton, Gopa Mitra, Sadia Khan and Heidi Wright for reviewing Chapter 6 and their suggestions for improving it.

Material for Chapters 5 and 7 was derived from a series of five focus groups that explored patients' and practitioners' perspectives of self care in summer 2005, organised, facilitated and reported by Matthew Critchlow on behalf of Health First in partnership with Lambeth and Southwark PCTs; we thank Dee Dulku, Charles Aina and Ros Band for their help in co-ordinating and facilitating the focus groups and providing input on the design and final report of that study.

Content throughout this book has been drawn and adapted from the following publications:

- Bayley H, Chambers R and Donovan C. *The Good Mentoring Toolkit for Healthcare*. Oxford: Radcliffe Publishing; 2004.
- Chambers R, Drinkwater C and Boath E. *Involving Patients and the Public* (2e). Oxford: Radcliffe Medical Press; 2003.
- Chambers R and Wakley G. *Clinical Audit in Primary Care: demonstrating quality and outcomes*. Oxford: Radcliffe Publishing; 2005.
- Chambers R, Wakley G, Iqbal Z and Field S. *Prescription for Learning: techniques, games and activities*. Oxford: Radcliffe Medical Press; 2002.
- Garcarz W, Chambers R and Ellis S. *Make your Healthcare Organisation a Learning Organisation*. Oxford: Radcliffe Medical Press; 2003.
- Mohanna K and Chambers R. *Risk Matters in Healthcare: communicating, explaining and managing risk*. Oxford: Radcliffe Medical Press; 2000.
- Wakley G and Chambers R. *Chronic Disease Management in Primary Care: quality and outcomes*. Oxford: Radcliffe Publishing; 2005.
- Wakley G, Chambers R and Gerada C. *Demonstrating your Competence 5: substance abuse, palliative care, musculoskeletal conditions, prescribing practice*. Oxford: Radcliffe Publishing; 2005.

About the Working in Partnership Programme (WiPP)

Workload is a key issue for primary care. This was confirmed in a national survey of general practitioner (GP) opinion in 2001 and later during the General Medical Services (GMS) contract negotiations. Survey responses demonstrated that there was a real need to address demand management. The consequences of not addressing GP workload would be widespread dissatisfaction and recruitment and retention problems.

At the GMS Contract roadshows, GPs complained about:

- excessive bureaucracy
- inability to spend sufficient time with patients
- some patients' unrealistic expectations
- undertaking consultations with patients who need not see a doctor.

The Working in Partnership Programme (WiPP) was established as part of the new GMS Contract arrangements, to address workload management in general practice.[1] Specifically, WiPP will identify, develop, signpost and mainstream effective ways to manage demand in general practice. This should create capacity in the primary care sector. Over the next two years, the programme will deliver a package of support that will enable practices and primary care trusts (PCTs) in England to:

- identify and analyse high-demand interventions as part of the development and delivery of effective services to manage those demands
- implement new ways of working, including new skill mix arrangements that have patients' support, which have safely and effectively demonstrated a reduced demand for services and/or more effective use of clinicians' time
- develop the public's capability to self care and take care of minor illness
- develop and deliver effective, integrated self care support resources for the public, largely provided by the community and voluntary sectors, and reduce reliance on mainstream NHS services
- simplify and improve the processes relating to the employment, training, development and retention of general practice managers, general practice nurses and health care assistants
- implement initiatives aimed at reducing bureaucracy.

The programme will focus on general medical practices, involving community pharmacists, local dentists and optometrists and their staff, allied health professionals and community health professionals.

Self care and the development of self care behaviours is a key work area for WiPP. WiPP supports four work programmes relating to the development of self care behaviours. These include:

- *Making Sense of Health:* support and resources for schools to embed health care messages with young people
- *Joining Up Self Care in the NHS:* a pilot scheme evaluating the benefits of an integrated self care model in Erewash PCT, Derbyshire
- *Self Care for Primary Healthcare Professionals:* this is a multidisciplinary training package and related resources for PCTs and practice teams
- *Self Care for People:* an initiative developing the role of a self care support co-ordinator in a PCT, developing a self care skills training course for local people.

Louise Jarvis

Reference

1 General Practitioners Committee/The NHS Confederation. *New GMS Contract. Investing in general practice.* London: British Medical Association; 2003.

Abbreviations

ABPI	Association of the British Pharmaceutical Industry
A&E	accident and emergency
AHP	allied health professional
BMI	body mass index
CAM	complementary and alternative medicine
CBT	cognitive behavioural therapy
CHD	coronary heart disease
CHIC	The Consumer Health Information Centre
COPD	chronic obstructive pulmonary disease
DAFNE	Dose Adjustment For Normal Eating
DESMOND	Diabetes Education and Self Management for Ongoing and Newly Diagnosed
DH	Department of Health
DiPEx	Database of Individual Patient Experiences
DPP	Developing Patient Partnerships
EBV	Epstein–Barr virus
EHC	emergency hormonal contraception
EMIS	Electronic Medical Information Service
EPP	Expert Patients Programme
FEV_1	Forced expiratory volume in 1 second
GABHS	group A beta-haemolytic streptococcus
GMS	General Medical Services
nGMS	new GMS (contract)
GP	general practitioner
HDL	high density lipoprotein
HbA_{1c}	haemoglobin A_{1c}
INR	international normalised ratio
KISS	keep it simple and short
KSF	Knowledge and Skills Framework
LDL	low density lipoprotein
LEAP	Learning and Employment Action Package
LES	local enhanced service
LMCA	Long-term Medical Conditions Alliance
LPC	local pharmacy committee
MAS	minor ailment scheme
MUR	medicines use review
NLP	neuro-linguistic programming
NPA	National Pharmaceutical Association
NPSA	National Patient Safety Agency
NSAID	non-steroidal anti-inflammatory drug

NSF	National Service Framework
OOH	out of hours
OTC	over-the-counter
P	pharmacy medicine
PAGB	Proprietary Association of Great Britain
PART	prevention, await resolution, relief of symptoms, toleration of symptoms
PCO	primary care organisation
PCT	primary care trust
PDSA	plan, do, study, act
PEST	political, economic, sociological and technological
PGD	patient group direction
PiP	Patient Information Publications
PLI	prescription-linked intervention
PMR	patient medication record
POM	prescription only medicine
PR	public relations
PSNC	Pharmaceutical Services Negotiating Committee
QOF	Quality and Outcomes Framework
RNIB	Royal National Institute of the Blind
RPSGB	The Royal Pharmaceutical Society of Great Britain
SIGN	Scottish Intercollegiate Guidelines Network
SIP	social inclusion partnership
SOP	standard operating procedure
SWAT	StaRNeT website assessment tool
SWOT	strengths, weaknesses, opportunities and threats
URTI	upper respiratory tract infection
WIC	walk-in centre
WiPP	Working in Partnership Programme

Part 1

Making self care happen

1

Supporting self care
Ruth Chambers

This chapter sets out the context, and what supporting self care means. It considers where we are now, how we have got here and where we want to go with self care.

To make self care work, both the public and professionals need knowledge and information (of facts and of where to find information), skills and motivation. The English public appears to be very interested in wanting to do self care, but a recent survey has shown that many lack the motivation, information and knowledge to adopt a healthy lifestyle and practise self care.[1] Box 1.1 captures the importance of the role of health professionals in primary care in encouraging and supporting patients' self care. The same survey concluded that:

> If professionals are to play an active role in self care, more work needs to be done with them to develop their role in supporting self care. Education and training are key, as change may require a culture shift from professionals being the principal providers of care and patients as passive recipients, towards more emphasis on preventative care, healthy lifestyle and patient involvement in their own care of minor, acute and long term conditions – with professionals providing a supportive, advisory, educational and skills training role.[1]

Support groups were found to have a role in providing advice, education and support – and self care support networks are part of the vision for the future.

Box 1.1: Key findings about the public's attitudes to self care
- More than half of those who have seen a care professional in the last six months say they have *not* often been encouraged to do self care, and one-third say they have *never* been encouraged by the professionals.
- Over three-quarters of the public agree that with guidance and support from an NHS professional they would be far more confident about taking care of their own health and wellbeing.
- Two-thirds of the public say they would be more confident in doing self care if they had support from people with similar health concerns or conditions.
- Awareness of patient organisations and voluntary agencies was low (68% of respondents were not aware of one).
- Few people say they have used NHS Direct in the last six months; however, they want to use the services more in the future.
- Family, friends and colleagues were the preferred source for self care information and support, after general practitioners (GPs) and nurses.[1]

The future for the NHS and support for self care

Emphasising self care by patients is a key strand in NHS delivery plans at all levels – strategically in the community services White Paper and locally in primary care trust (PCT) and practice development plans for all independent contractor practices.[2] Supporting self care for patients is part of the vision for development in the NHS through commissioning where responsibility is taken by a partnership operating between PCTs, general practice and local government, as a cost effective development that fits with patients' choice.[3]

The NHS must become 'as much a service to support health as to treat illness', where patients are empowered to take a more active self care role in maintaining or improving their health.[4] Table 1.1 describes some of the key messages in successive national policies about establishing self care in an integral way across the NHS and other government agencies.

There is a great deal of self care by members of the public occurring already, and lots of interest by the public in learning and reading what they can do for themselves (*see* Box 1.2).

Box 1.2: Key statistics describing activity around self care in England
- Over-the-counter medicine sales total £2 billion per year.
- Two-thirds of internet users have researched health issues online.
- Sales of consumer health magazines have grown at around 20% per year in the last decade.
- Around 1 million people are providing over 50 hours per week of unpaid care.[5]

What self care means – to the practice team

In future, local people should be:

> knowledgeable about the health and health care choices available to them . . . They should understand the links between lifestyle and health, and how to get support for changing their lifestyles when they need it.[4]

If people go to a pharmacy and discuss their symptoms, then the pharmacist and counter staff should be able to recommend that they self care, if appropriate, rather than consulting their GP. If they ring in or consult at the practice for a trivial reason, or return for a second opinion, then every member of the general practice team should give consistent health messages and advice as appropriate, all the time encouraging and supporting self care. Patients or people in the community can practise self care in their daily lives, provided they are able to trust and believe in the principles of self care and have the support or resources to be able to do so.

Figure 1.1 describes a real primary care team discussing how they define self care in their own words. It has been estimated that self-treatable disorders account for nearly 40% of GP time[5] – so there should be lots of opportunity for those working in primary care to encourage and support self care.[5]

Table 1.1: Examples of recent policy documents and reports following progress on self care (derived from www.pagb.co.uk and Department of Health (DH) sources)

Release date	Document	Extracts or key messages in document
1996	Towards a DH/NHS Strategy to Support Self Care[6]	'Do-it-yourself has been one of the major post-war consumer phenomena in the UK – many of us decorate our houses or maintain our cars with only occasional assistance from professionals. There are signs that a comparable revolution in health and wellbeing or "self care" may lie ahead. . . . The case for supporting self care is strong. There is substantial evidence to show that self care support leads to improvement in health outcomes and reduction in use of care services.'
2000	The NHS Plan. A plan for investment, a plan for reform[7]	'Most healthcare starts with people looking after themselves and their families in the home.' 'Professional training to include much more emphasis on self care, particularly for chronic conditions.' 'A wider range of over-the-counter medicines to be made available.'
2001	Securing our Future Health: taking a long-term view[8]	'Individuals will be responsible for more of their healthcare, either managing minor illnesses without the support of health care professionals or working with health care professionals taking a more active role in their own treatment.'
2001	The Expert Patient. A new approach to chronic disease management for the 21st century[2,9]	Expert Patients Programmes develop the confidence and motivation of people with a chronic illness, in using their own skills and knowledge to take effective control over their lives.
2003	Building on the Best. Choice, responsiveness and equity[10]	'Improving access to medicines . . . expanding the range of medicines which pharmacies can supply over-the-counter without a prescription . . . wherever it is safe to do so, make it simpler for patients to get treatments over-the-counter for conditions which until now have been regarded as strictly the preserve of the prescriber.'
2004	NHS Improvement Plan – putting people at the heart of public services[11]	'Expand the range of medicines the pharmacist can provide without a prescription. Promote minor ailment schemes where pharmacies can help patients manage conditions such as coughs, colds, hay fever, stomach upsets without a GP.'

Table 1.1: *Continued*

Release date	Document	Extracts or key messages in document
2004	*Delivering Choosing Health: making healthier choices easier*[12]	'For each of us, one of the most important things in life is our own and our family's health . . . this concern, and the responsibility that we each take for our own health, should be the basis for improving the health of everyone across the nation . . . [the White Paper] aims to inform and encourage people as individuals, and to help shape the commercial and cultural environment we live in so that it is easier to choose a healthy lifestyle.'
2004	*Better Information, Better Choices, Better Health – putting information at the centre of health*[13]	There are two key types of information people need: • 'general information available to all – about lifestyle options, care providers, diagnoses, conditions, self care and treatment options, standards of care etc • personal information – specifically on an individual's own condition, care options and possible outcomes.' We need to improve the relationship between patient and professional by: • 'mainstreaming communication training and development programmes for professionals to support a culture of shared decision making • developing a code of practice for professionals on good communication and information provision.'
2005	*Self Care – a real choice. Self care support – a practical option*[14]	'Self care includes the actions people take for themselves, their children and their families to stay fit and maintain good physical and mental health; meet social and psychological needs; prevent illness or accidents; care for minor ailments and long term conditions; and maintain health and wellbeing after an acute illness or discharge from hospital.'
2006	*Our Health, Our Care, Our Say – a new direction for community services* White Paper[2]	'One of the main ways [self care] can be delivered is through general practice, building on their responsibility for coordinating care . . . By 2008, we would expect everyone with a long term condition . . . to receive . . . self care support . . .'
2006	*Supporting People with Long Term Conditions to Self Care. A guide to developing local strategies and good practice*[3]	'We need to reach the stage where . . . professionals recognise that self care is a real choice and actively support the individual in this choice . . . Delivering effective self care support needs greater cooperation . . . to provide local solutions to embed supported self care into service delivery as a practical option.'

1 Individuals taking ownership of their own health, wellbeing and fitness
2 Educating patients about their responsibility and awareness of different approaches to self care
3 Providing types of self care support from within a range of practical options
4 Self care being at the centre of health care

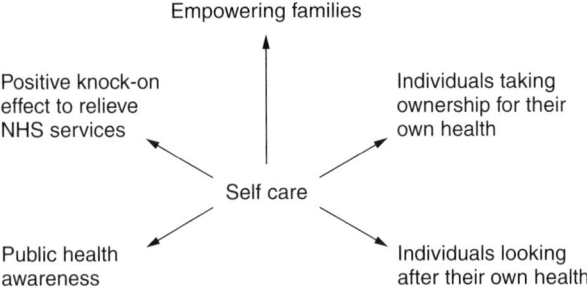

Figure 1.1: What self care means – to the practice team.

There is considerable antipathy about supporting self care in some practice teams or among some health professionals. Disaffected GPs might say: 'Good idea, but I once picked up a serious illness in a patient who came for something minor so you can't be too careful'. Or 'It's quicker to give a script than explain about alternatives and self care'. So professionals need to be encouraged to realise the benefits of self care – such as by spelling out that time spent advising on and treating minor conditions could be better focused on the more major health problems included in the Quality and Outcomes Framework.[5,15]

Establishing an integrated strategy for supporting self care in practice

Initiatives to encourage self care in the practice are more likely to be successful if they are fully integrated into the delivery of general medical services by the primary health care team. A self care support strategy should be integral to all other strategies and development plans in a PCT or practice – and appropriate for the local population. It should avoid merely transferring dependence from one professional (e.g. a GP) to another in a different setting (e.g. a pharmacist).

Self care approaches should be interesting and meaningful to patients and the public, to encourage changes in their behaviour. Erewash PCT, for example, focused on three key areas: minor ailments, chronic disease (e.g. asthma) and the presentation of coronary heart disease. They set up the Pharmacy First initiative whereby patients can use the pharmacy instead of their GP practice. They held seasonal campaigns – linking in pharmacies, and focusing on hay fever, coughs and colds, etc. The initiative broke down barriers between GPs and pharmacists, to build trust and consistency and create a team approach to supporting self care.[15] The PCT ran self care skills training for people with asthma, associated with their Expert Patients programme. They also provided a simple visual coronary heart disease (CHD) risk self-assessment 'wheel' in a range of community locations and linked that to further information on CHD.

An integrated self care support strategy should be based on the following principles:[15]

- integration means that self care fits into all strands of the PCT operations – public health, commissioning, primary care and communications – led from the top with investment and commitment
- use patient-relevant strategies
- use language and communication that people understand
- a self care support resource should be diverse and engaging – so people will have real options to choose from
- make the most of opportunistic times when people will be maximally willing to receive information about self care, e.g. antenatal care, after a heart attack, etc
- primary health care teams are pivotal to success or failure of any local initiative – it is easy to underestimate the time, professional barriers and effort required for practice teams to institute a new approach – such as promoting self care
- use marketing and public relations (PR) companies to get the messages across to the public – this will make the most of the time and investment by the local NHS in supporting self care
- conceive self care as something people can do all the time as part of a lifetime habit. Everyone self cares, some do it better than others. Think what we have to do to help people self care even better. Most self care is done subconsciously. Self care for a long term condition may be done consciously to start with until it becomes a habit
- the whole workforce should receive self care skills training, so that they understand why and how to enable self care by patients – from counter staff in pharmacies to top people in the PCT
- communication campaigns from central government, the media, and any local ones should be co-ordinated
- PCTs need to communicate with the community and find out what they want – self care support networks and resources in different languages should be developed to really make self care happen by individualising the approach according to the nature of their community.

Health inequalities and self care

Self care support for patients and the public is one ingredient in improving the health of the community and reducing health inequalities. Other health inequalities are unavoidable, being due to genetic and biological differences between people. Some inequalities arise from differences in opportunity, in access to services (health and social care, education, leisure etc), in their environment and material resources, as well as in lifestyle behaviour such as diet, exercise and smoking. Poor living and working conditions resulting from poverty, little education and inadequate housing also contribute to health inequalities.[16]

People who have these disadvantages may potentially benefit most from strategies to encourage and support them to practise more self care. But they are often the most challenging groups of people to help. They may be more difficult to access, and more resistant to change. Someone who is aware of the benefits of change, trusts the health professionals advising them and is used to making autonomous decisions, is more likely to be helped to change, than someone who is instinctively mistrustful of authority figures, has low self confidence and had limited benefits from the education system in the past. Any general practice team or PCT has to come up with a very wide-based strategy that caters for all types of people in a way that redresses these inequalities to promote self care effectively. They will need well-designed resources matched to a person's needs and way of life.

Health and social services support for self care

Making self care effective will require increasing the capacity, confidence and efficacy of patients and the public for self care. There is also need to build on social capital in the community. The ideas in Box 1.3 describe actions that health and social care services can take to boost the chances that individuals in their community will practise self care for themselves or those they care for.[17] Most of these ideas can be incorporated into everyday general practice with good planning and resources.

Box 1.3: Methods of health and social services support for self care
- Appropriate and accessible advice, information and campaigns on lifestyle issues to change behaviours (such as physical activity, healthy eating, other behaviours to sustain wellbeing and prevent ill health) and to change the care of minor, acute and long term conditions
- Health education (such as adult health skills and health literacy programme)
- Self care skills training, for example through the Expert Patients Programme
- First aid training in schools for children
- Health promotion in schools: exercise, diet, learning to say 'no' to smoking, drugs, alcohol and other unhealthy practices
- Self-diagnostic tools, self-monitoring devices and self care equipment
- Multi-media, multi-lingual self care information and skills training materials
- Individualised care plans
- Support networks of people with experience and memory of healthy living and of caring for minor, acute or long term conditions
- Active participation of the public locally and nationally in the formation and implementation of relevant local and national government policies and programmes
- Education of the public and practitioners to change their attitudes and behaviours towards self care
- Training of practitioners in when and how to use approaches to support self care
- Work to develop partnerships between care professionals and the public to enhance shared care and for patients and the public to become co-producers of their care

Moving from medical care to self care in the future

A review of the long term future of the NHS highlighted the potential of self care as a key factor in the change of demand for care services.[8] Wanless predicted a switch of 2% of GP activity to pharmacists, and a reduction of 17% in outpatient attendances among people practising self care. In his scenario the general public become fully engaged in improving their health, for example through better lifestyles and more self care. Some research highlighted in the report suggested that visits to GPs could decline by over 40%.

Many people with long term conditions are already involved in self care actions. Chronic disease currently costs the UK government £12 billion per year in disease management and lost earnings.[18] In one national telephone survey, 79% of people with diabetes were self-monitoring their diabetes, though far fewer of those with hypertension or lung disease were self-monitoring their condition. Education is a key component in empowering patients to take care of their own chronic disease, but the capacity to self manage health and health care is least evident among people with poor health.[19]

Promoting health and wellbeing through self care support

You can target health education at whole populations, e.g. giving advice on the prevention of depression to everyone you see. Alternatively, you can target high-risk groups, e.g. giving advice on the prevention of depression to elderly people with precipitating causes such as bereavement.

The Health Development Agency evolved a resource for improving the health and wellbeing of people in mid-life (aged 50–65 years; *see* Box 1.4).[20] This age range is recognised as a period of mid-life transition when people address various issues including their health; there are opportunities to increase life expectancy and preparing for a healthier older age.[12]

Box 1.4: Taking action at local level: a resource for improving health and wellbeing in mid-life

The resource provides information and suggestions about:[20]

- relating to regional and national policy initiatives
- identifying mid-life needs within a locality
- identifying partners
- building a case for action
- identifying which models to use and the evidence available
- developing ways to evaluate initiatives.

When undertaking health promotion, GPs and other health professionals need strategies to encourage people's individual action (empowerment) rather than use coercion or blame, as the essential nature of health education is that it is voluntary.

People do try self care before engaging with the NHS. But they may abandon this too soon believing that their 'symptoms are persisting', not necessarily because their home remedy is no longer relieving their symptoms, but being unsure whether their symptoms are due to something more serious. Their presentation to the doctor or triage nurse offers the opportunity to have a self care aware consultation; their own home remedy, herbal or over-the-counter medicine, complementary therapy or remedy can continue to provide relief.

Creating a safe self care culture

Understanding of safety and risk by the NHS in general as well as by those people practising self care is another facet in the creation of a self care culture. Ensuring that the care patients receive is safe and effective is at the heart of everything that the NHS and social services do. The better your systems are at identifying and managing risk, the safer your practice will be. The National Patient Safety Agency (NPSA) has a practical checklist (*see* Box 1.5) that a PCT or practice team could use to underpin the safety of their self care support strategy and practice.[21]

Box 1.5: Seven steps to patient safety – in relation to supporting self care

1 *Build a safety culture*: so you minimise risks to patients whilst supporting self care.
2 *Lead and support your staff*: establish a clear and strong focus on patient safety throughout your PCT/practice.
3 *Integrate your risk management activity*: develop systems and processes to manage your risks and identify and assess things that could go wrong – eliminate inadequate training, or encourage an incompetent person to self care.
4 *Promote reporting*: ensure staff can easily report incidents relating to self care that have gone wrong, in a central log.
5 *Involve and communicate with patients and the public*: communicate openly with, and listen to, patients – do not thrust self care at them.
6 *Learn and share safety lessons*: encourage staff to learn from any incident arising from supporting self care and communicate this to each other.
7 *Implement solutions to prevent harm*: embed lessons through changes to practice, processes or systems relating to the promotion of self care.[21]

In conclusion

Self care by patients is central to the vision for reform in the NHS. The Department of Health intends that:

> the healthcare system will become more proactive in working with patients to enable them to manage and protect their own health in the long term. Local practices will have incentives to provide locally based health improvement and health protection services. They will be able to use their budgets to invest in such services which could be provided by the local PCT or by private or voluntary sector providers, or by a combination of these. Patients for their part, empowered by more and better information and able to choose from a range of services, will be in a stronger position to manage their own health and wellbeing. Tackling inequalities in health will become more important, as it will ensure that more people can benefit from good health.[22]

References

1. Department of Health. *Public Attitudes to Self Care Baseline Survey*. London: Department of Health; 2005.
2. Department of Health. *Our Health, Our Care, Our Say – a new direction for community services*. White Paper. London: Department of Health; 2006.
3. Department of Health. *Supporting People with Long Term Conditions to Self Care. A guide to developing local strategies and good practice*. London: Department of Health; 2006.
4. Hewitt P. *The Nation's Health and Social Change*. Discussion Paper. London: The New Health Network; 2005.
5. Colin-Thomé D. *The Policy Drivers for Self Care*. Presentation to 8th annual Self Care Conference 29 September 2005, London.
6. Department of Health. *Towards a DH/NHS Strategy to Support Self Care*. Working Paper. London: Department of Health; 1996.
7. Department of Health. *The NHS Plan. A plan for investment, a plan for reform*. London: Department of Health; 2000.
8. Wanless D. *Securing our Future Health: taking a long-term view*. London: HM Treasury; 2002.
9. Department of Health. *The Expert Patient. A new approach to chronic disease management for the 21st century*. London: Department of Health; 2001.
10. Department of Health. *Building on the Best. Choice, responsiveness and equity*. London: Department of Health; 2003.
11. Department of Health. *NHS Improvement Plan – putting people at the heart of public services*. London: Department of Health; 2004.
12. Department of Health. *Delivering Choosing Health: making healthier choices easier*. London: Department of Health; 2005.
13. Department of Health. *Better Information, Better Choices, Better Health – putting information at the centre of health*. London: Department of Health; 2004.

14 Department of Health. *Self Care – a real choice. Self care support – a practical option.* London: Department of Health; 2005.

15 Pringle M. *Managing Everyday Healthcare – implementing an integrated self care strategy at PCT level.* Presentation to 8th annual Self Care Conference 29 September 2005, London.

16 Department of Health. *Tackling Health Inequalities: status report on the programme for action.* London: Department of Health; 2005.

17 Dost A. *Further Towards a Self Care Support Strategy.* Leeds: Economics and Operational Research Division, Department of Health; 1998.

18 Alder J. *Incidence of Chronic Disease Set to Soar unless we Manage it Better.* London: Chronic Disease Working Party, Cass Business School; 2005. www.cass.city.ac.uk

19 Ellins J and Coulter A. *How Engaged are People with their Healthcare?* Oxford: Picker Institute Europe; 2005.

20 National Institute for Health and Clinical Excellence. *Taking Action at Local Level: a resource for improving health and wellbeing in mid-life. Part 1: Developing local strategies.* London: NICE; 2005. www.nice.org.uk

21 www.npsa.nhs.uk

22 Department of Health. *Health Reform in England: update and next steps.* London: Department of Health; 2005.

2

What we know about the practice and impact of self care

Ruth Chambers

This chapter describes the scope of self care in the UK and considers what we know from recent work in the field about its impact.

Self care is the basic level of health care in any society.[1] In the UK, self care comprises an estimated 80% of all care episodes. Figure 2.1 shows the relationship of self care to professional care, and demonstrates how professionals and the public are co-producers of care.

Self care is a continuum, starting from the individual responsibility people take in making daily choices about their lifestyle, and risk taking. This may be in their work, travel and hobbies, and other aspects of their everyday lives. Next along the continuum, Figure 2.2 shows the self care of ailments without and with assistance from health professionals such as pharmacists, GPs or practice nurses. Shared care follows – by health professionals together with their patients, as individuals cope with long term health conditions and acute health problems. Ultimately on the right hand of the continuum there is 100% professional care with little or no opportunity for self care in the immediate episode, e.g. complex co-morbidities, compulsory psychiatric care or major trauma or illness – until the start of recovery when self care can emerge again.

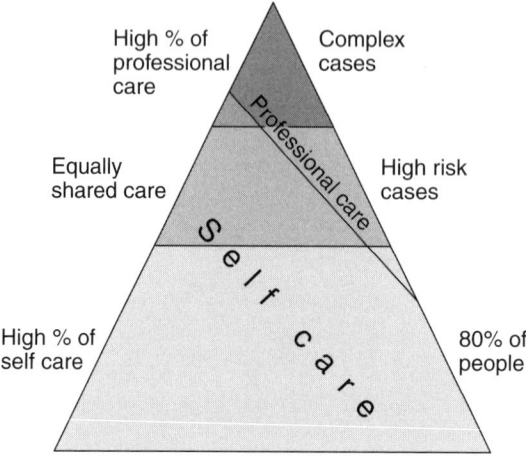

Figure 2.1: The health care pyramid.

What we know about the practice and impact of self care

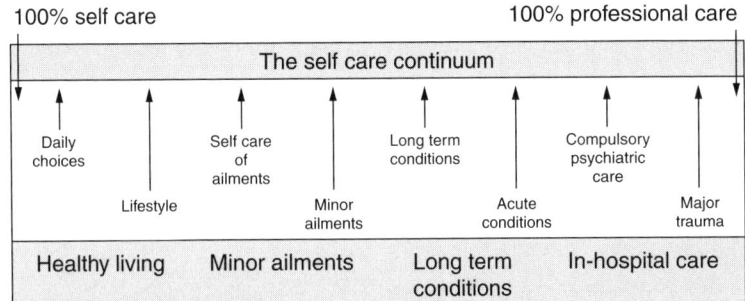

Figure 2.2: The self care continuum.

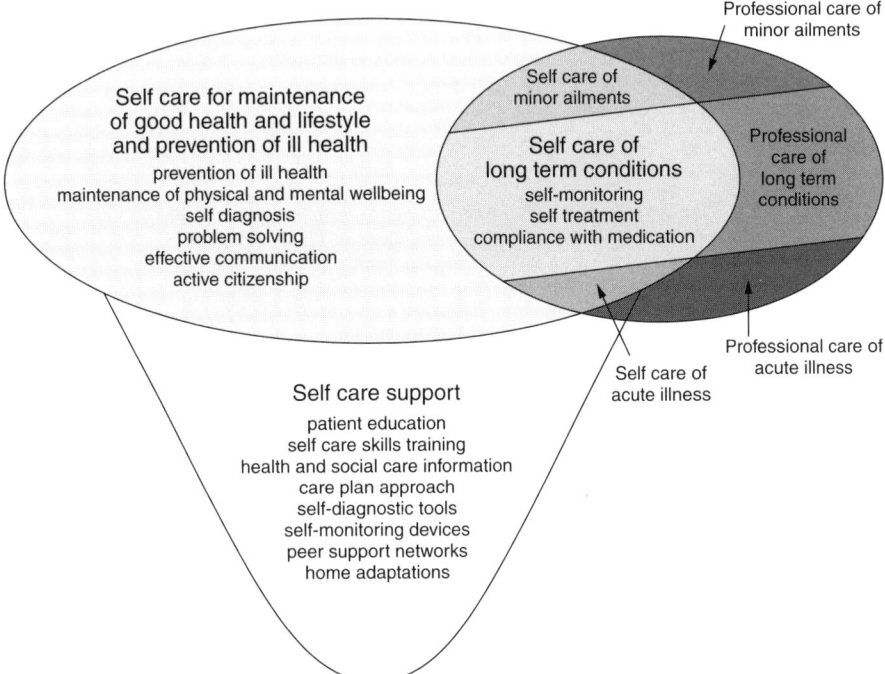

Figure 2.3: Self care support for maintenance of good health and lifestyle, and prevention and care of ill health (courtesy of Ayesha Dost, Department of Health).

Figure 2.3 maps the various approaches to self care, from the achievement and maintenance of good health and a healthy lifestyle to the prevention of ill health and minimising symptoms from minor illness. The figure also introduces the inter-relationship between the promotion of health in the community through social care, outside the primary care setting.

Components of self care

The aims of promoting self care among your patients or the local population are to encourage individual people to:

P: **P**revent the condition developing
A: **A**wait resolution of the symptoms
R: use self care skills for **R**elief of symptoms
T: learn to **T**olerate symptoms that do not resolve or cannot be reasonably alleviated.[1]

The size of each PART quadrant in Figure 2.4 will depend on the specific level and range of self care skills for a particular condition.

P Prevent the condition developing	A Await resolution of the symptoms
R Use self care skills for Relief of symptoms	T Learn to Tolerate symptoms that do not resolve or cannot be reasonably alleviated

Figure 2.4: The PART model to illustrate pathways for self care.

Enhance the level of self care skills of individuals and self care support provided by the NHS by considering each component. Push the boundaries of self care to the maximum that is safe for your patients or the general public, and affordable in terms of resources such as time and capacity of primary health care professionals.

Some self care support approaches will focus on one of the quadrants. Others may have more than one component in the total intervention. The case study in Box 2.1 combines **P**revention of worsening asthma using preventive therapy more effectively and by smoking cessation, with **R**elief through better use of medication.

Box 2.1: Case study: proactive self care support for people with asthma

Fifty practices in 25 PCTs are participating in 'Asthma Care', a proactive telephone outreach service to support self care. A nurse contacts individual patients in a series of regular calls to discuss their asthma and related issues. Smoking cessation advice is also given, as is explanation of the importance of preventer therapy, and where reliever therapy fits in. Overall, around one-third of patients did not have an action plan for their asthma. Patients were referred to their asthma nurse or GP where needed. An evaluation was conducted with 150 patients who had completed the programme and reported: better understanding of their asthma (86%); improvement in their asthma (69%); better compliance with preventer medicine (39%); reduced amount of reliever medicine taken (40%). Patients felt they had time to discuss their questions and had confidence they could raise other issues.[2]

The case study reported in Box 2.2 describes **T**olerance and **A**waiting resolution as well as **R**elief of children's minor ailments. Involving the family and carers is important in promoting self care. Families have a strong influence on someone's use of health services and health seeking behaviour.[3,4]

Box 2.2: Case study: education and advice on children's minor ailments

Sure Start and four local pharmacies on an estate in Hull are collaborating to make greater use of pharmacies as health advice centres. The aim is to increase parent education on health issues in under-three year olds in an under-doctored area. Parents register with a local pharmacy for advice on children's minor health problems that they would otherwise have consulted the GP about. Simple information leaflets are distributed on the six ailments covered by the scheme: temperature/aches/pains; stuffy nose; colic; nappy rash; diarrhoea/sickness; teething; dry skin. Pharmacists can supply medicines free of charge for five of the six ailments. So far, no medicine has been supplied in 10–15% of cases. In roughly half of these, the pharmacist's view is that advice is sufficient and for the rest they think that referral for medical advice is necessary.[2]

Some conditions lend themselves to self care more than others. Problems such as back pain or sore throat are likely to get better anyway without any medical management or treatment. At the same time, people need information about the occasional serious aspect of their illness that requires medical attention. The 'red flags' in back pain, which if undetected and treated as an emergency can lead to permanent paralysis, or the very occasional sore throat that turns out to be a quinsy, require a safety net. Chapters 10 to 13 contain in-depth illustrative patient pathways covering back pain, asthma, cough and sore throat, and demonstrate how the four components of self care – prevention, await resolution, relieve symptoms and tolerance – apply to each condition. Look at Box 2.3 to think more about selecting appropriate types of self care support intervention.

Box 2.3: Gaining maximum impact from self care support intervention

A review of qualitative research on self care concluded that:[5]

a number of factors need to be considered when devising health care interventions for managing demand better. These include an assessment of the meaning of the disease to the person so that self care information can be designed in a way that fits people's prior beliefs and lifestyles. Timing and

> the stage in a person's illness career are also important factors to consider when designing effective self care support interventions. Social interaction and the impact of significant others may affect whether or not a self care regime is followed, and autonomy and control are also relevant to designing acceptable self care strategies.

There are many innovative practical examples of self care support across all health settings. In a recent review no examples of a whole systems approach to self care across a health economy were found.[2]

Educational interventions

People are capable of making informed choices and undertaking self care all along the continuum of Figure 2.2 from their increased understanding and motivation gained by educational interventions. A review of medical self care interventions concluded that:[5]

> education in self care decision making and practices can produce significant effects in terms of health care utilisation and cost reductions.

It seems more worthwhile to focus educational campaigns on targeted individuals who have reason to benefit from self care. The consensus among health education researchers seems to be that behaviour change is unlikely to result from mass communication campaigns alone.[6] One evaluation of a cold/'flu self care public education campaign, for example, resulted in no changes in people's beliefs, attitudes, acquisition of new health practices or self-reported visits to the doctor.[6]

The successful educational intervention may be just a simple explanation, targeted at the right person at an opportune time. In one study concerning children with earache, a brief explanation by the doctor to the parent about the inadvisability of using antibiotics resulted in 50% decrease in antibiotic use.[7] Hopefully that learning would continue for further episodes, resulting in fewer future consultations with a doctor for earache.

Poor patient understanding about their disease is believed to impede appropriate self care. Finding the right educational interventions that will have a long term impact on enabling self care and improving health outcomes in chronic disease is difficult. Any educational initiatives need to be designed with an awareness of the complexity of people's social and cultural experiences and attitudes typical of their community.[8,9] When considering the content or delivery of any intervention, remember who the target audience is and what specific barriers there may be to it being effective.[10]

Consider how to match the type of educational intervention to a particular person to optimise its impact.[11] Your information could be in the form of a book or leaflet, audiotape, interactive online resource, quiz, self-assessment checklist, poster, video, digital patient story or peer with similar condition. Ensure that the person you are trying to educate with such information materials really does have the disease it relates to and has not been misdiagnosed or is assuming that they have a condition they have not got. That is difficult when information or education is simply made available for members of the general public or patients in general – but the material should be explicit and clear.

Use educational interventions that include specific information about inappropriate and harmful treatments too, and symptoms that could generate mistreatment – not just the simple guidance you hope to deliver about straightforward self care. It is easy to assume that people have basic knowledge which in reality they do not possess and that could undermine their ability to self care.[12]

Educational interventions are more likely to be cost effective if targeted at 'high risk' patients. For health education targeted at frequent users of health services, with conditions such as high blood pressure, diabetes, heart disease, back pain, it was found that slightly fewer consultations were recorded with a doctor in the subsequent six-month period combined with a little improvement in their health risk scores.[13] Another educational intervention involving people with Parkinson's disease resulted in fewer visits to the doctor and fewer symptoms.[14]

Just as with the Expert Patients Programme (EPP) in England (*see* p. 106), another study of a self management education programme has reported a reduction in pain and use of health services for people with chronic arthritis.[15,16]

Experience with self care health books is mixed. One American study considered the effects of distributing a series of seven self care brochures with home remedies and guidance on the appropriate use of health services for a common cold, sore throat, headache, fever, 'flu, earache and back care.[17] The majority of recipients 'liked or strongly liked' the information and most kept the brochures at home. Health service use was unaffected and the researchers concluded that 'educational programmes are more effective in raising awareness than in changing behaviour during the initial stages of an intervention'. It is likely that to achieve a reduction in use of health services requires:

ongoing and repetitive educational messages . . .

patients who feel more responsible for self care of simple health conditions who begin to consider taking a more active role in health improvement in other lifestyle related behaviours too.[17]

In another study nearly half of the 1967 patients in one practice who were given a self care book had consulted it. Those with health problems were more likely to have looked at it. Of those who had looked at the book, 60% reported that the book made them more likely to deal with a problem themselves, and 40% replied that they were less likely to consult the practice. However, the study found that there were *no* differences in consultation rates between those who had, or had not read the book they had received, or between those who received the book or others who had not had a copy of the self care book.[18]

Box 2.4 describes a selection of other educational programmes and their likely benefits.

> **Box 2.4:** Examples of educational interventions linked to promotion of self care
>
> - Effects of educational and psychosocial interventions for adolescents with diabetes mellitus: these had small to medium beneficial effects on various diabetes-related outcomes.[19]
> - A whole systems approach to self management which included a self care guidebook for people with inflammatory bowel disease + physicians trained in patient-centred care + negotiated written self management plan. This trial resulted in fewer hospital visits without change in the number of primary care visits, fewer symptom relapses, and most patients liked the new system.[20]
> - Information leaflets from voluntary groups or charitable organisations can enable people to take care of themselves. For example, the Arthritis and Rheumatism Council issues practical advice on management of rheumatic disease, including a handout on knee pain self management which stresses the importance of type and duration of exercise.[21]
> - A study involving people with hypothyroidism showed:
>   brief intervention with an educational booklet has no influence on thyroxine adherence or health in patients with primary hypothyroidism. These findings do not support the routine distribution of health educational materials to improve medication adherence.[22]
> - Intergenerational projects whereby older people support and challenge youngsters can improve older people's self worth, and thus health. Active ageing is the focus of the charitable organisation, the Beth Johnson Foundation.[23]
> - Self help promotion clinics are another type of intervention that aim to empower people to improve their health and wellbeing. One study of a self help mental health clinic found that the combination of self help materials and individually tailored programmes of self help by a therapist allowed patients to self care, and limited the face-to-face therapist input of traditional services.[24]
>
> Other examples are given in a self care compendium of practical examples.[2]

For every research study with positive findings there are probably many more that are unpublished as they have no positive findings. Consider too how long the participants in any study were followed up, and whether the impact of any educational intervention lasted for more than a few months.

It appears it is not sufficient to simply distribute educational materials. You also need to engage with the recipients to generate more impact on their behaviour from the intervention; or share decision making to enable individuals to help themselves.[25] A review of self help books available for depression illustrated the importance of engaging patients, maybe in cognitive behavioural therapy over time, running alongside their reading of the book.[26] You need to consider the costs incurred by such health professional support in enabling self care.

An intensive educational intervention given to people with asthma to encourage self management of their medication resulted in fewer consultations, days off work and courses of antibiotics. There were better quality of life scores with good adherence to agreed self management plans. But this was an intensive and therefore costly programme involving participants learning about lung anatomy and physiology, asthma and its causes, the effect and purpose of medication and the principles of self management, from specially trained nurses. They also received physio-therapeutic counselling.[27]

The *Joining Up Self Care* initiative in Erewash PCT has several strands, enabling people to take steps towards self care. As well as valuable information, an individual can use an aid to self assess their risks of heart disease based on their lifestyle and family history. They can obtain a lifestyle pack that matches their self-assessed level of risk from a local pharmacy or by making a free telephone call.[28]

There are a number of other very useful structured education programmes for people with diabetes. In the DAFNE (Dose Adjustment For Normal Eating) programme, participants with type 1 diabetes learn how to adjust their insulin dose to suit their choice of food.[29] With DESMOND (Diabetes Education and Self Management for Ongoing and Newly Diagnosed), participants with type 2 diabetes identify their own health risks and set their own specific behavioural goals.[30,31]

Self care guides

In future, people's individual electronic health records should be linked with self care information and self care plans. The public already has access to national resources available for self care such as the NHS Direct range of services including the NHS Direct Healthcare Guide, NHS Interactive on digital TV, NHS Direct Online and algorithms (*see* page 94) or the self care booklet produced by the Developing Patient Partnerships (DPP).[32–34] The internet site BestTreatments developed in association with NHS Direct is based on *Clinical Evidence* and has resources for patients, as well as health professionals.[35,36] Similarly, *Prodigy* contains information sheets that can be printed off for individual patients.[37]

The example in Box 2.5 is of a guidebook for promoting patient participation in the care of ulcerative colitis.

Box 2.5: Features of a successful self help guidebook

Patients with ulcerative colitis were involved throughout the process of developing a guidebook on the condition. Information was designed to empower patients and allow them to participate in making informed choices about their medical and surgical care. Patients wanted the content to: be positive about life with a chronic disease, explain the rationale behind treatment, give facts and figures about likely outcomes, and be updatable.[38,39]

Self care of long term conditions

People report that self management of their long term condition puts them in control of their lives. An individual's involvement in self management is likely to fluctuate over time depending on how much time and importance they give to it.[40] Self management skills training in the early stages of a condition should help to prevent the onset of complications and further disability.[41]

Elements of self management support for people with long term conditions include:

- patient education
- patient psychosocial support
- self management assessment
- self management resources
- collaborative decision making
- guidelines available to patients.

Most NHS trusts have tried various forms of self care support for people with long term health conditions. These might be in the form of outreach support for conditions like asthma, educational programmes such as for diabetes or preventing falls, promotion of healthy lifestyles, for example through walking or by forming self care support networks. Some PCTs produce their own local health magazines. An effective approach to the care of people with long term conditions requires a system that works across the various settings of health and social care as an integrated system.

There is interest in the UK in the Kaiser Permanente approach from the US.[42] The Kaiser programme encourages self management by patients through lifelong learning. Patients are encouraged to take more responsibility for their own health. Kaiser provides patient education material on its website (www.kaiserpermanente.org) for patients to access. Patients are educated in hospital to take care of their own health after discharge.

UK Pfizer Health Solutions helps people with long term conditions to become more active in taking care of their own health. The company works with NHS commissioning bodies to provide tailored services to meet the needs of local populations, drawing on experience from the US. A review of the US health system concluded that:

> case and disease management programmes in which support for self management is a central feature should be developed in every PCT.[43]

NHS policy documents on care of people with long term conditions have emphasised the contribution of self care support. The long term conditions National Service Framework (NSF) aims to transform the way that health and social care services support people to live with long term neurological conditions.[44] The NSF features supporting self care around the needs and choices of individuals including health promotion.

Although enthusiasm is growing for self management programmes for people with long term conditions, there is conflicting information about their effectiveness and what their essential components are. A meta-analysis that considered 780 published studies concluded that:

> self management programmes for diabetes mellitus and hypertension probably produce clinically important benefits . . . osteoarthritis self management programmes do not appear to have clinically beneficial effects on pain or function.[45]

Self-monitoring of blood pressure may give a truer estimate of usual blood pressure than readings by a doctor in the surgery and may save time for health professionals. However, there is evidence that blood pressure measured by patients is inaccurate in as many as 50% of patients.[46] Another study enabled patients to take their own blood pressure, but at the general practice rather than in their homes, and initiate a consultation with their doctor or nurse if their blood pressure was repeatedly above target levels. This style of self-monitoring resulted in small but significant improvements of blood pressure at six months, which were not sustained after a year.[47] The researchers concluded that practice-based self-monitoring of blood pressure is feasible; the self-monitoring was well received by patients, their anxiety did not increase, and there was no appreciable additional cost.

Several studies have indicated that patient self management may improve the quality of oral anticoagulant therapy.[48,49] In one study, patients measured their international normalised ratio (INR) using the CoaguChek S every two weeks, or more frequently if required, for six months. They adjusted their own warfarin dose on the basis of their INR using the algorithm provided. The researchers concluded that:

> in the majority of suitably trained patients, the quality of oral anticoagulant therapy achieved through self management is comparable to that obtained by self testing patients managed by a specialised hospital anticoagulation service.[48]

The second study over 12 months drew similar conclusions, and noted that patients with poor control before the study showed an improvement in control through self management.[49]

Experience of self management to date indicates that a whole systems approach is needed that improves information given to and shared with patients, improves access to services and encourages health professionals to adopt a more patient-centred approach.[50] Self care information on its own is of limited effectiveness. When this whole systems approach was adopted with guided self management of ulcerative colitis, patients preferred it to traditional outpatient care; there was earlier treatment of relapses and fewer follow-up visits to health services.[51] Open access to health services may fit better with patients' self management of their condition and everyday routines, roles and responsibilities.[52] Lay-led self management may be more effective than that which is professionally led (fitting with the ethos of the Expert Patients Programme[15]) when targeted at minority groups so that lay leaders may overcome cultural and language barriers. One such initiative had some success when lay tutors led a six week programme of three-hour sessions for Bangladeshi adults living in London, known to have diabetes, arthritis, respiratory or cardiovascular disease – although moderate uptake and attendance limited the benefits gained.[53]

Using assistive technologies

Assistive technologies include a broad range of technologies such as home adaptations, as well as newer technologies such as email and text messaging. Some devices such as blood glucose monitors or nebulisers contribute to patients' self care. Email and text messaging are cheap and fast and are limited by patient preferences, as is use of the internet as a health resource.[40,54] Other devices range from sophisticated ones such as telemedical monitors to simple ones that are readily available in the high street, such as pedometers.[55]

Self care support networks

The evidence for the benefits of lay-led self care networks, some of which may also be called 'self help groups', is still scant.[56] They are a potentially important method of delivering self care interventions for people with specific conditions and/or their carers. Many groups provide unstructured support with variable quality of self care materials. A review of the effectiveness of self help mutual aid groups in America found positive outcomes such as reduced psychiatric symptoms, less use of professional services, enhanced coping skills, increased life satisfaction and shorter hospital stays.[57] Box 2.6 relays some tips for anyone setting up a local self care support network.

Box 2.6: Encouraging local development of self care support networks
- Don't reinvent the wheel: get a starter pack from a group that already exists.
- Find a suitable meeting place and time.
- Publicise and run your first community meeting.
- Meeting tasks: be clear about the purpose – perhaps provision of emotional support, practical information, education, and advocacy. Set out basic guidelines such as about confidentiality. Define the membership, meeting format, people's roles and responsibilities, and the use of professionals. Exchange contact details.
- Start with a small project and work up to more difficult tasks.[58]

Self care support provided by pharmacists

Chapter 6 contains many examples of self care support by pharmacists and their teams. Relatively simple interventions can make a big difference. A one-hour educational and medicines management visit by a community pharmacist which emphasised self care, medications and screening processes for complications, resulted in improved diabetic control in a study involving 80 patients. Teamwork between the pharmacist and health professionals in the general practice team was key.[59]

Some PCTs have tried out Pharmacy First (www.erewash-pct.nhs.uk). Box 2.2 described the collaboration between Sure Start and four pharmacies in Hull in making greater use of pharmacies as health advice centres.

Can we afford to promote self care?

Some examples included here have demonstrated that supporting self care can result in tangible benefits to people's health and thus cost savings to the NHS and society in general, as healthier people can work harder and more effectively, for longer. While specific and reliable information about the cost effectiveness of the various types of self care is limited, the promotion of self care has been recognised as an important aspect of managing demand.[60] However, for any significant effect on demand in primary care, multifaceted approaches are required at all points, from avoidance of first contact with health services to possible referral to secondary care. The various components of an integrated self care support resource and the entire range of self care interventions must be considered when advising and supporting patients.[61]

The Wanless review suggested that in general for every £100 spent on encouraging self care, £150 worth of benefits can be expected in return.[62] In a systematic review of self help treatments for anxiety and depression in primary care, none of the eight studies included had data on long term clinical benefits or cost effectiveness.[63] A systematic review of the clinical and cost effectiveness of patient education models for adults with types 1 and 2 diabetes, for instance, found 24 studies of such education; but only two of these reported on the cost effectiveness of their educational intervention.[64] The trial of self-monitoring in hypertension found that self-monitoring did not cost significantly more than usual care.[47] A trial of a guidebook offering self help information plus a self help group meeting resulted in a 60% reduction in primary care consultations, and costs were reduced by £73 per year.[65] For the present, self care support may be developed and promoted in the hope that it will result in affordable benefits and be cost effective. Evidence suggests that

> intervening at the community level is potentially more powerful or at least more cost effective than interventions at individual level[66]

unless the interventions are targeted at high risk individuals.

References

1. WONCA (World Organization of Family Doctors). *The European Definition of General Practice/Family Medicine*. Barcelona: WONCA Europe; 2002.
2. Department of Health. *Self Care Support: a compendium of practical examples across the whole system of health and social care*. London: Department of Health; 2005.
3. Dean K. Self-care responses to illness: a selected review. *Social Science and Medicine*. 1981; **15A**: 673–87.
4. Cardol M, Groenewegen PP, de Bakker DH et al. Shared help seeking behaviour within families: a retrospective cohort study. *British Medical Journal*. 2005; **330**: 882–4.
5. Kemper DW, Lorig K and Mettler M. The effectiveness of medical self-care interventions: a focus on self initiated responses to symptoms. *Patient Education and Counselling*. 1993; **21**: 29–39.
6. Vingilis E, Brown U, Koeppen R et al. Evaluation of a cold/flu self-care public education campaign. *Health Education Research*. 1998; **13**: 33–46.

7 Pshetizky Y, Naimer S and Shvartzman P. Acute otitis media – a brief explanation to parents and antibiotic use. *Family Practice.* 2003; **20**: 417–19.

8 Sanchez CD, Newby LK and McGuire DK. Diabetes-related knowledge, atherosclerotic risk factor control, and outcomes in acute coronary syndromes. *American Journal of Cardiology.* 2005; **95**: 1290–4.

9 Stone M, Pound E, Pancholi A *et al.* Empowering patients with diabetes: a qualitative primary care study focusing on South Asians in Leicester, UK. *Family Practice.* 2005; **22**: 647–52.

10 Garlick W. *Patient Information. What's the prognosis?* London: Consumers' Association; 2003.

11 Jenkinson D, Davison J, Jones S *et al.* Comparison of effects of a self management booklet and audiocassette for patients with asthma. *British Medical Journal.* 1988; **297**: 267–70.

12 Green K. Common illnesses and self-care. *Journal of Community Health.* 1990; **15**: 329–38.

13 Fries JF and McShane D. Reducing need and demand for medical services in high-risk persons. A health education approach. *Western Journal of Medicine.* 1998; **169**: 201–7.

14 Montgomery EB, Liebermann A, Singh G *et al.* Patient education and health promotion can be effective in Parkinson's disease: a randomised controlled trial. *American Journal of Medicine.* 1994; **97**: 429–35.

15 www.expertpatients.nhs.uk

16 Lorig KR, Mazonson PD and Holman HR. Evidence suggesting that health education for self-management in patients with chronic arthritis has sustained health benefits while reducing health care costs. *Arthritis and Rheumatism.* 1993; **36**: 439–46.

17 Terry PE and Pheley A. The effect of self-care brochures on use of medical services. *Journal of Occupational Medicine.* 1993; **35**: 422–6.

18 Platts A, Mitton R, Boniface D *et al.* Can self-care health books affect amount of contact with the primary health care team? *Scandinavian Journal of Primary Health Care.* 2005; **23**: 142–8.

19 Hampson SE, Skinner TC, Hart J *et al.* Effects of educational and psychosocial interventions for adolescents with diabetes mellitus: a systematic review. *Health Technology Assessment.* 2001; **5(10)**.

20 Kennedy A, Robinson A, Nelson E *et al.* A randomised controlled trial to assess the impact of a package comprising a patient-orientated, evidence-based self-help guidebook and patient-centred consultations on disease management and satisfaction in inflammatory bowel disease. *Health Technology Assessment.* 2003; **7(28)**.

21 Arthritis and Rheumatism Council (ARC). *An Exercise in Knee Pain Self-management.* Chesterfield: ARC. www.arc.org.uk/about_arth/rdr5.htm

22 Crilly M and Esmail A. Randomised controlled trial of a hypothyroid educational booklet to improve thyroxine adherence. *British Journal of General Practice.* 2005; **55**: 363–8.

23 www.bjf.org.uk

24 Lovell K, Richards DA and Bower P. Improving access to primary mental health care: uncontrolled evaluation of a pilot self-help clinic. *British Journal of General Practice.* 2003; **53**: 133–5.

25 Coulter A. What do patients and the public want from primary care? *British Medical Journal.* 2005; **331**: 1199–201.

26 Anderson L, Lewis G, Araya R *et al*. Self-help books for depression: how can practitioners and patients make the right choice? *British Journal of General Practice*. 2005; **55**: 387–92.

27 Lahdensuo A, Haahtela T, Herrala J *et al*. Randomised comparison of guided self management and traditional treatment of asthma over one year. *British Medical Journal*. 1996; **312**: 748–52.

28 Erewash PCT. *Welcome to the Erewash Heart-to-Heart Assessment; Welcome to your Green Lifestyle Pack*. Ilkeston: Erewash PCT; 2005.

29 www.dafne.uk.com

30 www.desmond-project.org.uk

31 Department of Health. *Structured Patient Education in Diabetes*. London: Department of Health; 2005.

32 Banks I. *The NHS Direct Healthcare Guide*. Oxford: Radcliffe Medical Press; 2000.

33 www.thomsonlocal.com

34 Banks I. *Better Health at Home and at Work. A self-care guide*. London: Developing Patient Partnerships; 2005.

35 www.besttreatments.co.uk

36 www.clinicalevidence.com

37 www.prodigy.nhs.uk

38 Kennedy AP, Robinson AJ, Thompson DG *et al*. Development of a guidebook to promote patient participation in the management of ulcerative colitis. *Health and Social Care in the Community*. 1999; **7**: 177–86.

39 Kennedy AP and Rogers AE. Improving patient involvement in chronic disease management: the views of patients, GPs and specialists on a guidebook for ulcerative colitis. *Patient Education and Counselling*. 2002; **47**: 257–63.

40 Corben S, Rosen R. *Self-management for Long-term Conditions*. London: King's Fund; 2005.

41 Matrix Research and Consultancy. *Learning Distillation of Chronic Disease Management Programmes in the UK*. London: Modernisation Agency, Department of Health; 2004.

42 Ham C, York N, Sutch S *et al*. Hospital bed utilisation in the NHS, Kaiser Permanente and the US Medicare programme: analysis of routine data. *British Medical Journal*. 2003; **327**: 1257–60.

43 Dixon J, Lewis R, Rosen R *et al*. *Managing Chronic Disease. What can we learn from the US experience?* London: King's Fund; 2004.

44 Department of Health. *The National Service Framework for Long-term Conditions*. London: Department of Health; 2005.

45 Chodosh J, Morton SC and Mojica W. Meta-analysis: chronic disease self-management programs for older adults. *Annals of Internal Medicine*. 2005; **143**: 427–38.

46 Turnbull SM, Magennis SP and Turnbull CJ. Patient self-monitoring of blood pressure in general practice: the 'inverse white-coat' response. *British Journal of General Practice*. 2003; **53**: 221–3.

47 McManus RJ, Mant J, Roalfe A *et al*. Targets and self monitoring in hypertension: randomised controlled trial and cost effectiveness analysis. *British Medical Journal*. 2005; **331**: 493–6.

48 Gardiner C, Williams K, Mackie IJ et al. Patient self-testing is a reliable and acceptable alternative to laboratory INR monitoring. *British Journal of Haematology*. 2005; **128**: 242–7.

49 Fitzmaurice DA, Murray ET, McCahon D et al. Self management of oral anticoagulation: randomised trial. *British Medical Journal*. 2005; **331**: 1057–9.

50 Kennedy A, Rogers A. Improving self management skills: a whole systems approach. *British Journal of Nursing*. 2001; **10**: 734–7.

51 Robinson A, Thompson DG, Wilkin D et al. Guided self management and patient directed follow-up of ulcerative colitis: a randomised trial. *The Lancet*. 2001; **358**: 976–81.

52 Rogers A, Kennedy A, Nelson E et al. Patients' experiences of an open access follow up arrangement in managing inflammatory bowel disease. *Quality and Safety in Health Care*. 2004; **13**: 374–8.

53 Griffiths C, Motlib J, Azad A et al. Randomised controlled trial of a lay-led self-management programme for Bangladeshi patients with chronic disease. *British Journal of General Practice*. 2005; **55**: 831–7.

54 Mead N, Varnam R, Rogers A and Roland M. What predicts patients' interest in the Internet as a health resource in primary care in England? *Journal of Health Service Research Policy*. 2003; **8**: 33–9.

55 Department of Health. *Supporting Self Care – A Practical Option: Diagnostic, monitoring and assistive tools, devices, technologies and equipment to support self care*. London: Department of Health; 2006.

56 Department of Health. *Evidence from UK and International Studies on Self Care Support Initiatives*. London: Department of Health; 2005.

57 Kyrouz EM, Humphreys K and Loomis CL. A review of research on the effectiveness of self help mutual aid groups; expanded and updated. In: White BJ, Madara EJ (eds). *American Self-Help Clearinghouse Self-Help Group Sourcebook* (7e) New Jersey: American Self-Help Clearinghouse; 2002.

58 www.bhrm.org/Guide.htm

59 Chloe HM. Proactive case management of high risk patients with type 2 diabetes mellitus by a clinical pharmacist: a randomised controlled trial. *American Journal of Managed Care*. 2005; **11**: 253–5.

60 Chapple A and Rogers A. Self-care and its relevance to developing demand management strategies: a review of qualitative research. *Health and Social Care in the Community*. 1999; **7**: 445–54.

61 Gillam S and Pencheon D. Managing demand in general practice. *British Medical Journal*. 1998; **316**: 1895–8.

62 Wanless D. *Securing our Future Health: taking a long-term view*. London: HM Treasury; 2002.

63 Bower P, Richards D and Lovell K. The clinical and cost-effectiveness of self-help treatments for anxiety and depressive disorders in primary care: a systematic review. *British Journal of General Practice*. 2001; **51**: 838–45.

64 Loveman E, Cave C, Green C et al. The clinical and cost-effectiveness of patient education models for diabetes: a systematic review and economic evaluation. *Health Technology Assessment*. 2003; **7(22)**.

65 Robinson A, Lee V, Kennedy A *et al.* A randomised controlled trial of self-help interventions in patients with a primary care diagnosis of IBS. *Gut* 2006; **55**: 643–8: 10.1136/gut.2004.062901. http://gut.bmjjournals.com/cgi/reprint/55/5/643.pdf

66 Hibbard J, Greenlick M, Jimison H *et al.* The impact of a community-wide self-care information project on self-care and medial care utilisation. *Evaluation and the Health Professions.* 2001; **24**: 404–23.

3

Getting organised for supporting self care as a primary care organisation

Ruth Chambers

This chapter describes how you can get organised in a primary care organisation to design a strategy and implementation plan in relation to supporting self care. The outcome should be a culture where supporting self care is integral to all the PCO's functions; and the workforce promotes and supports self care in effective ways as part of their everyday work.

Stage 1: getting commitment – developing your vision

First ensure that you are committed to embracing the comprehensive strategy that Wanless envisaged, to

> incorporate a wide range of approaches and models of self care, including finding ways of providing funding, information, facilities, equipment and technology to support its development.[1]

Identify a minimum number of champions in your PCT to promote self care and to join up as a working group. They will need to interact with key committees and individuals in the PCT whose support and commitment are essential to enable self care support interventions or evolve a self care culture. Make the case for a PCT strategy and implementation plan – as in the algorithm of Figure 3.1 (adapted from the Faculty of Public Health).[2] Or use the Working in Partnership training programme (WiPP) to run an action learning set (*see* Box 3.1).

Box 3.1: Using the WiPP multidisciplinary training package in a PCT

Rather than a traditional working group run as part of PCT core business, you could use the WiPP training programme to work out your approach as a PCT to supporting self care, and implementing your plans. The WiPP website has instructions on running the action learning group and the facilitator's handbook.[3] Use the electronic versions of the 21 tools (*see* Figure 3.1) reproduced in Part 3 of this book. Log your progress online.

The training programme cannot be prescriptive, as participating PCTs will be at varying levels of expertise and have different capacity in their evolution of a self care culture. PCTs already have their own traditions as to how they plan and establish new initiatives, and the training package takes account of these. The exact nature of self care interventions and activities you prioritise will depend on local resources, the nature of your local population, the educational environment and enthusiasm of your local workforce.

We propose a minimum of three facilitated learning and development sessions with intervening associated work being undertaken by individuals and sub-groups or committees. Some PCTs may organise more facilitated meetings – exact arrangements will depend on local preferences and capacity.

While a draft PCT strategy is developing, or has been evolved and agreed, those in lead or responsible positions in the PCT should involve general practice teams and other individuals and teams relevant to self care, such as patients and pharmacists, to revise and finalise the strategy and action plan. General practice teams and others involved in providing self care will then be encouraged and facilitated to mirror or adapt the strategy and actions relating to self care for their own teams in their workplaces.

A PCT might consider the following options:

1 running an action learning set in the PCT – around eight leads and champions who work together over a period of time (e.g. a year), meeting regularly (e.g. two-monthly) under the guidance of a facilitator (not necessarily present at all meetings)

or

2 a working group to establish self care support within the PCT, with minuted meetings and review of actions, to evolve and implement a self care support strategy; with a chair who is a champion for self care. This is likely to span a minimum of a year. Sub-groups may develop particular elements of the integrated self care support resources between meetings.

Who should you involve?

Include one or more of the champions in the following development areas who will assume leadership and take responsibility for:

- overall strategy/development
- co-ordination of the strategy action plan, learning lessons and subsequent change
- co-ordination with other PCT initiatives and priorities and other stakeholders e.g. out of hours and emergency care, long term conditions, Expert Patients Programme (EPP), minor ailments schemes, the Quality and Outcomes Framework (QOF) in GP practices, pharmacy and dental contracts, local delivery plans, colleagues in secondary and tertiary care sectors or social services, community and voluntary groups
- finance and other resources
- education and training – facilitation of learning across the PCT
- clinical governance – patient safety, risk
- changing workforce
- special interests e.g. health promotion, disadvantaged groups, patient and public involvement
- monitoring and sustainability – cost effective review
- clinical pathways and subsidiary protocols: to include self care support components

- public health – interface with self care
- communication and dissemination/public relations
- liaison between discipline groups: e.g. general medical practice teams, community staff (district nurses, school nurses, health visitors, allied health professionals), pharmacy teams, PCT management, health trainers, community matrons.

Start with Tool 1 which explains how to undertake a force-field analysis and consider the positive drivers in your PCT for deciding to draw up and implement a strategy for supporting self care. You can derive many of the positive factors from the evidence for the effectiveness of self care described in Chapter 2. On the opposing side will be the negative factors you should take into account before committing to the strategy. Include them in your implementation plan in considering how to overcome barriers to change.

Having decided at PCT board level to proceed to draw up a strategy on promoting self care, use Tool 2 to help you work through the stages of drawing up the strategy and setting priorities. You might find Tool 3 useful to run an analysis of the strengths, weaknesses, opportunities and threats (SWOT) relating to establishing a culture of self care support in your PCT. Key steps are described in Box 3.2 and in more detail in Figure 3.1.

Box 3.2: Developing a self care support strategy in a PCT
- Agree the need for a self care support strategy
- Develop a committed working group
- Define clear and realistic aims and objectives
- Appoint a project lead
- Ensure the right people are involved and key stakeholders are with you
- Identify and plan adequate resources
- Maintain stakeholder commitment and motivation in a working group[3]

There are three key challenges for PCTs in supporting self care for people with long term conditions:

1. developing the skills of professionals to support self care – some health professionals may mistakenly interpret self care as compliance with medical instructions
2. improving the provision of information about long term conditions and the local services available
3. increasing the flexibility of service provision to fit in with patients' other commitments.[4]

The vision will capture the aspirations of your PCT. Your vision needs to be embedded in reality otherwise there is a danger of it becoming more of a hallucination! A clear, shared vision of the future will help shape change. The person responsible for communication needs to get everyone on board. Your vision should be underpinned

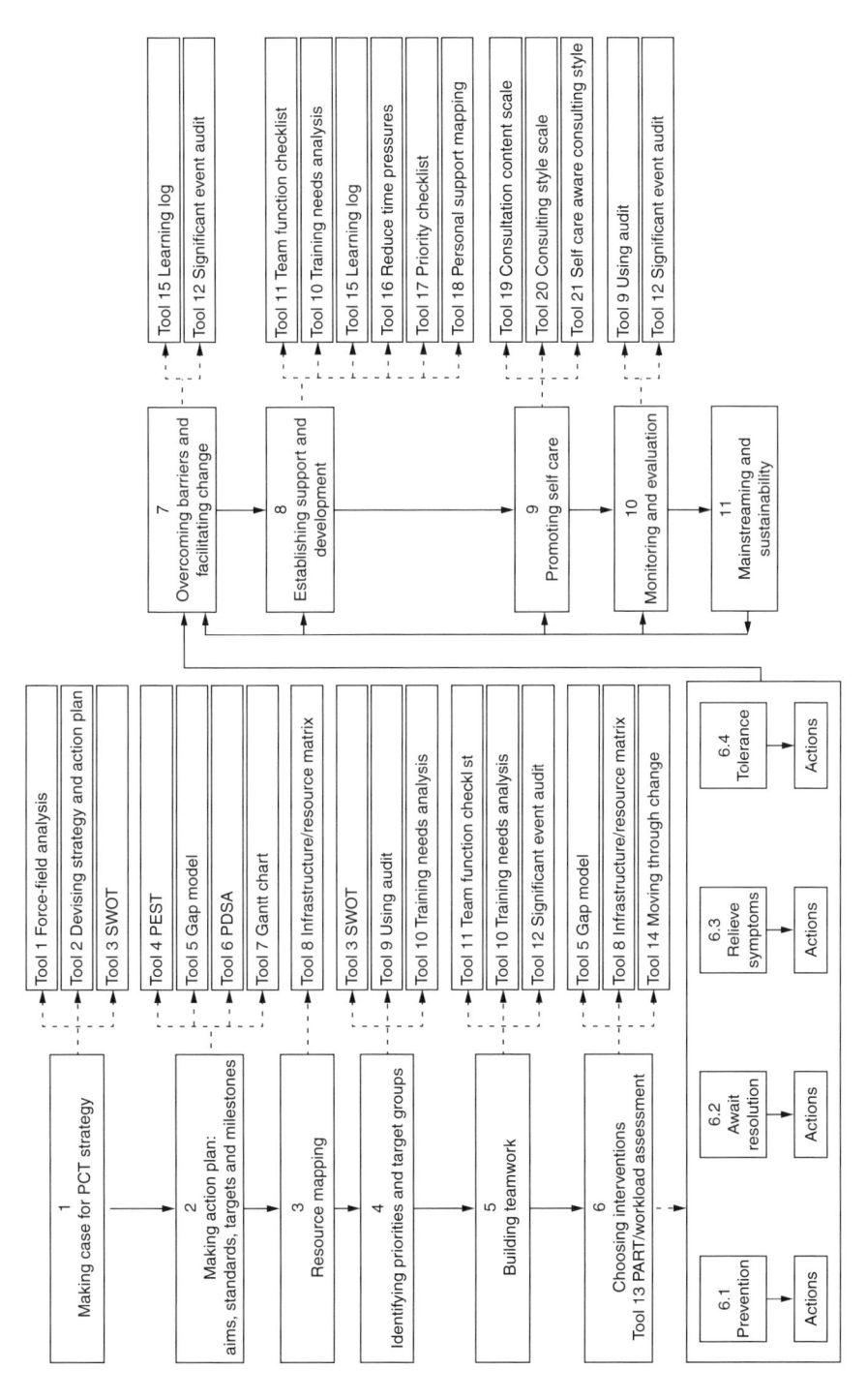

Getting organised for supporting self care as a primary care organisation

Figure 3.1: PCT perspective for establishing an integrated resource to support self care.

by the principles and attitudes underlying your values. Self care must be safe care and promoted for all in an equitable way.

Making your action plan

Consider the political, economic, sociological and technological (PEST) factors that will influence your PCT's action plan, as in Tool 4. Or undertake a gap analysis considering where you are now (with unstructured self care support initiatives) and where you want to be (an evolving culture of self care support rolled out as an integrated resource across the PCT) – *see* Tool 5. Refer back to the vision you described at the first meeting of your working group when defining your aims.

As a next stage, undertake a self care needs analysis to feed into Tool 4 and/or Tool 5 of your local population including minority groups. Consider the:

- perceptions and expectations of your population
- perceptions of health professionals providing the services – PCT employed staff and those in independent contractor practices
- perceptions of commissioning managers and those responsible for providing services, based on available data about the size and severity of health issues for your population and known inequalities
- priorities of the PCT and population linked to national, regional or local priorities.[5]

The 'plan, do, study, act' (PDSA) approach of Tool 6 may be the model that helps you to construct your action plan. Map out a timetable for your prioritised actions – adapting the example Gantt chart in Tool 7 to include your actions and milestones.

Resource mapping

Think about resources you already have for supporting self care within your PCT and its constituent practices, and those you need. The infrastructure and resource matrix of Tool 8 should help you map out your current resources, and then plan what extra resources you need. This includes all kinds of resources – knowledge and skills and attitudes of your workforce, self care materials, other local stakeholders or partners in your self care initiative, your information resources or those freely available nationally, etc.

Remember you are not building up an integrated self care support resource on your own. Harness the enthusiasm of general practices, pharmacists and dentists who are promoting self care. Work with social care, community and voluntary groups and share their resources too. Work on creating a healthier community for your local population, with other local organisations who share that responsibility. A self care support strategy can run through your joint initiative. There are several resource packs and toolkits you could use to guide you on a community-wide strategy in general, or specifically focused on a health issue such as reducing the prevalence of obesity.[2,6,7] Box 3.3 includes some top tips on creating effective partnerships.

> **Box 3.3:** Top tips for effective partnerships
>
> Effective partnerships in relation to supporting self care should have:
> - shared vision and common priorities
> - a strategic planning framework – themes, population groups, areas, settings
> - strategic partnership structure and accountability arrangements
> - champions and leaders at strategic and operational levels
> - co-ordinated needs assessment and community involvement
> - cross-cutting commissioning arrangements
> - flexible use of resources – staff, money, time, facilities
> - a co-ordinated approach to mainstreaming initiatives
> - common local targets and indicators
> - partnership learning and staff development.[8]

Commissioning self care support: for your priorities and target groups

The commissioning section of your action plan will rely on the data you have gathered, the evidence for self care support (*see* Chapter 2), information from your working group and workforce, evaluation (*see* Chapter 9) and knowledge management.[9,10] Self care commissioners need to:

- understand their population, knowing its needs and wants
- understand self care and its norms, benchmarks and evidence
- understand how to make change
- have good processes in the PCT which enable decisions to be made quickly and securely.

Use Tool 3 to undertake a SWOT analysis and/or Tool 9 to carry out audits of your current performance or application of resources relating to self care, to help you gather data about your baseline position, in respect of your patient population and any target groups. This should identify or reaffirm your priorities – the type of self care support and patient groups you will focus on.

Devising an education and training framework for the PCT in relation to the promotion of self care

Promotion of effective self care support as a common activity by health professionals will only happen if the workforce has the right knowledge and skills and a positive attitude to self care, as well as practical options for providing support. Your working group should consider agreeing an appropriate education and training programme for all health staff to meet the requirements of the PCT in establishing self care support (*see* Figure 3.2), before finalising the PCT's self care support strategy and action plan. Start at the bottom of Figure 3.2 at the baseline and work upwards through the figure.

1. The baseline includes your starting point as regards the budget, numbers of staff, their skill base and the extent and quality of education and training activities

available relating to self care. Think about knowledge, skills, and positive attitudes and behaviour.
2. The next stage is the preliminary identification of the education and training needs of the workforce you are planning for across your PCT. This should take account of gaps in the baseline resources you identified, the short and longer term visions of development for your PCT, and how national, regional and local workforce planning strategies affect you. Anticipate workforce trends in designing your education and training programme. Otherwise delays will occur while you recruit and train new staff if you need additional personnel such as a PCT trainer to lead on supporting self care.
3. The constraints of your budget will start to bite as you begin to plan your education and training programme and turn your preferred vision into your affordable vision. Budget limitations, the workforce's willingness to co-operate with the programme, and the need to make the programme relevant to service needs, other competing priorities and local issues, will all influence its design. The nature of your education and training programme relating to self care will be influenced by:
   - the historical provision the workforce are used to and may be willing to take up (e.g. going to lectures)
   - their preferences for particular modes of delivery (team members learning together and putting learning into action)
   - current fashions (self care in this case; type of delivery such as e-learning)
   - pressure from local champions or special interest groups like public health, for their favourite causes (e.g. encouraging healthy lifestyles, or the 'Back in work' campaign).
4. Once the affordable vision is agreed at a planning stage, provision can be mapped out. This should include meeting the needs of all the PCT/practice workforce involved in respect of:
   - generic knowledge and skills e.g. interacting effectively with patients and the public
   - uni-professional education and training e.g. special roles for reception staff or pharmacists
   - multiprofessional provision whenever appropriate and practicable (to learn together around a protocol for particular conditions where self care is viable)
   - managerial or organisational education and training for those with roles associated with evolving a safe culture of self care across the PCT.

Appraisal and evaluation of the skills, knowledge, attitudes and competence of the workforce involved should be a regular feature of any education and training programme, with feedback about achievements and gaps in provision at all stages in the cycle. Recommend Tool 10 for individuals in your working group or workforce at large, to help them identify their training needs – to be addressed by the PCT's (or their employer's) education and training strategy and implementation plan.

Getting organised for supporting self care as a primary care organisation

```
                    ┌─────────────────────────────────────────────┐
                    │ Appraisal of workforce:                     │
                    │  • numbers: skill mix, range, seniority     │
                    │  • skills: range, depth, appropriateness    │
                    │  • performance: minimum standards, best practice │
                    └─────────────────────────────────────────────┘
                                      ▲
          ┌───────────────────────────────────────────────────────────┐
          │ Re-skilled or adapted workforce promotes self care within limited resources │
          └───────────────────────────────────────────────────────────┘
                                      ▲
```

Appropriate and affordable education and training provision

| uni-professional specialist education and training in respect of role | multi-professional education and training focused on self care | generic education and training: • management/change • organisational planning • workforce planning |

Minimum awareness and possession of core skills e.g. teamwork, good communication with patients, shared decision making, motivating to healthy state

Planning meetings/networking/leadership

pressure groups → ← historical patterns

current resource limitations → Affordable vision ← skill mix

lay/citizens' views → ← additional funds

- gap analysis: what are we trying to do, what resources have we got, what resources do we need, how do we close those gaps?
- what is needed for short term plans and long term vision?
- manpower planning (skills and numbers)
- individuals' and organisation's performance

Education and training needs

- funds: trust allocation, other such as linked to regeneration
- personnel: numbers, skills – generic
  – core
  – specific
- educational provision: quantity and quality and providers

Baseline resources

Budget ← competing priiorities

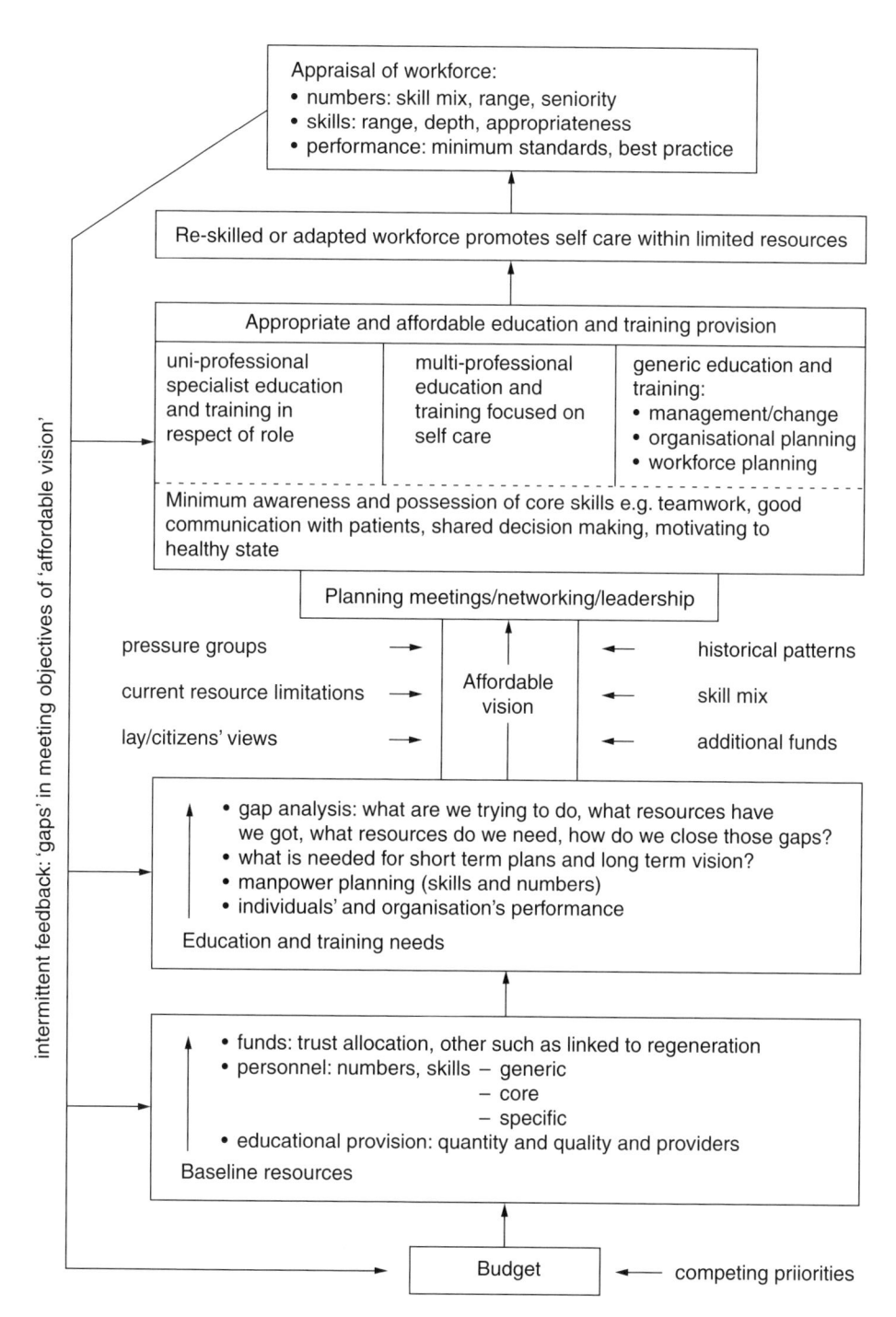

(left side label: intermittent feedback: 'gaps' in meeting objectives of 'affordable vision')

Figure 3.2: Framework for the education and training programme for a PCT (or practice) in relation to supporting self care for patients and the local community.

Building teamwork

A team may be clinical – in your PCT or in a general practice; health professionals have to work together and with patients. It may be organisational – as with your working group on the self care support strategy and implementation. Team members need to respect the skills and contributions of other team members. All should be clear about their roles and responsibilities.

You will depend on the teams in your PCT and out on the frontline in composing and implementing your self care support strategy. Try out Tool 11 on your immediate teams to check how well they are functioning. If there are any crises or complaints, undertake a significant event audit as in Tool 12.

Choosing interventions

The interventions you select will depend on your priorities and target groups. Tool 13 may be more pertinent to general practice action planning. It assesses the clinical and organisational workload generated by a variety of example health conditions, then considers what can be done in respect of prevention, awaiting resolution, relieving symptoms and toleration for those conditions (see p. 16 and Chapters 10–13). As a PCT you might work with several practices and support them using Tool 13. Then you could collate what help and support practice teams need, and apply that resource on a PCT-wide basis, addressing your whole patient population. Examples include:

- those responsible for public health and health promotion in your PCT might work with other partners on aspects of prevention
- a minor ailment scheme with pharmacists (see p. 84)
- enhanced services with general practices that cover self-monitoring of anticoagulant therapy (see p. 23)
- extending the EPP initiative (see p. 106)
- creating more local smoking cessation or exercise on prescription schemes[11]
- appointing and supporting health trainers to support people in the local community with greatest needs[12]
- marketing better health to the community with social services and educational bodies as in the Slough project[13]
- focusing on people with long term conditions with the highest risks of health care usage in primary care, or of admission to hospital[14,15]
- focusing on more organisational interventions, helping practice teams to gain new skills or move through change (see Tool 14).

Go back to Tool 3 to carry out a SWOT analysis or Tool 5 to undertake a gap analysis if that helps you to select priority interventions. Read through documents that encapsulate the learning of other PCTs who are already supporting self care and are actively promoting it.[16,17] Consider resource implications of your chosen interventions using Tool 8.

Lastly

Many a health service strategy gathers dust on the bookshelf for the reasons listed in Box 3.4. Include actions to ensure that your self care support strategy and implementation plan is widely welcomed and gains general ownership.

Box 3.4: When a strategy goes wrong ... it may be because:

It is not read or understood
Once a strategy has been produced it needs to be seen, read and understood by the target audience. Careful thought needs to be given as to how the message should be communicated to key movers and shakers.

It is too vague and woolly
An implementation plan with targets and milestones is essential.

It is too prescriptive
A strategy which is too detailed and lacks flexibility may not meet local needs and then fails.

It lacks ownership
An essential element of strategy development should be to engage key players; this includes patients, carers and the wider public.

There are unexpected events
Unexpected events, such as a new government initiative, can blow a strategy off course. The strategy should be flexible to enable it to adapt to new circumstances.

It is launched at the wrong time
The timing can be wrong for an otherwise perfect strategy – it may be ahead of its time or too late. You can develop a strategy and wait for the right time for its implementation.

Of the financial implications
With many competing priorities for scarce health service resources, a strategy should assess the financial implications and see that appropriate resources are secured.

Stage 2: keeping going

Look back at Figure 3.1 for where you are on your route to establishing a self care culture across your PCT with effective self care resources and interventions applied by a willing workforce. Adopting a developmental approach should encourage staff, rather than issuing 'top down' directives that are resented by staff and difficult to implement. Otherwise, frontline staff will view self care as just adding to their workload, and not part of demand management.

Everyone working on, or associated with, the self care strategy should be clear about the goals, individuals' roles and responsibilities, timetabled programmes for improvements, and standards of performance required.

Overcoming barriers and facilitating change

The most commonly perceived barriers to supporting self care initially in the *Joining Up Self Care* initiative are described in Box 3.5.

> **Box 3.5:** Barriers to extending self care
> - The most frequently mentioned barriers were time and resources.
> - Patients' lack of knowledge about possible services and sources of advice was frequently mentioned. There were some sceptical or negative views from health professionals about patients' ability and/or willingness to take up self care.
> - Negative attitudes and lack of knowledge and skills of health professionals in relation to self care were recognised. Awareness of opportunities to support self care during consultations was lacking across all the professional groups.
>
> (Holmes J. *Joining Up Self Care – baseline health professional research*. Personal communication, 2005)

Encourage health professionals who have attended initial training on self care aware consultation techniques, or are considering supporting self care, to keep a learning log during their everyday practice, as in Tool 15. Or suggest they undertake a significant event audit relating to their promotion of self care support succeeding or failing as in Tool 12. Encourage practice teams to think about what worked out well, or what got in the way using Tools 12 and 14 or any other Tools. They should come up with solutions they can sustain to overcome barriers and move towards supporting self care as part of their everyday practice.

Establishing support and development

As a PCT you need to work closely with practice teams of GPs and other independent contractors to help them build momentum for supporting self care. Look back at Chapter 2 to see the conclusions about successful self care support – i.e. the whole systems approach that is needed.[18] You need well-educated health professionals to be able to communicate ideas on self care to individual patients consulting them. Patients themselves need to be offered the information they want and need. The spoken word needs to be reinforced – by guided self management, personal care plans, online resources, etc. The PCT should promote parallel activities at community level and in schools.[19]

The education and training you provide, signpost or commission should:

- match health professionals' learning needs (*see* Tool 10)
- support good practice teamworking (*see* Tool 11)
- encourage reflection on performance and learning from experience (*see* Tool 15)
- promote efficient working and service provision so that there is time to promote self care during consultations (*see* Tool 16)

- help practice teams to assess self care as a priority for learning and service development (*see* Tool 17).

Mirror this range of encouragement and support you will be extending to practice teams within your PCT employed workforce too.

Supporting self care

Your actions to support self care will be a continuation of the self care interventions you selected earlier. Encourage the application of Tool 13 workload assessment in general practices or discuss the range of self care support initiatives described in Chapter 2 and match them with your population's needs. The experience of the *Joining Up Self Care* initiative described in Box 3.4 shows the importance of encouraging good patient-centred consultation techniques in your health professional community – so advocate Tools 19 and 20 for your workforce to assess their consultation skills and style. You could use Tool 21 as a core component of a workshop on self care skills training for your PCT workforce.

Lastly, remember that promoting self care will be tough. Anything new that requires such significant change in knowledge, skills, attitudes and behaviour, will be difficult and may seem overwhelming to people already working under pressure. Encourage your workforce and health professional community to look after themselves too. Tool 18 is a good start, for individuals to map out the types and extent of support in their own lives, and see which sources of support can be boosted.

Stage 3: monitoring and evaluation

Evaluation is an essential component of any programme or service. Incorporate it into your action plan from the beginning, matched to your vision and aims. Time and effort spent on evaluation should be in proportion to the activity that is being evaluated. Keep it as simple as possible to avoid wasting resources on unnecessarily bureaucratic evaluation. Use Tools 9 and 12 to undertake audits of the self care outputs and activities being generated by your self care support strategy and its implementation. Look at Chapter 9 for more on evaluation.

Mainstreaming and sustaining a self care culture in your PCT

Your strategy and action plan is directed at establishing a culture of supporting self care, rather than perceiving this as a time-limited project. Activities and milestones should reflect the mainstreaming and sustaining of achievements you expect. Re-assess your priorities and resource needs as you gather data evaluating your progress to date. You will be moving in a circular fashion to re-examine barriers to progress and facilitate further change – as in the algorithm of Figure 3.1.

References

1 Wanless D. *Securing our Future Health: taking a long-term view*. London: HM Treasury; 2002.

2 Swanton K. *A Toolkit for Developing a Local Strategy to Tackle Overweight and Obesity in Adults and Children*. London: Faculty of Public Health; 2005.

3 Working in Partnership Programme. *Self care in Primary Care – a new way of thinking.* London: Department of Health; 2005. www.wipp.nhs.uk

4 Corben S and Rosen R. *Self-management for Long-term Conditions*. London: King's Fund; 2005.

5 Cavanagh S and Chadwick K. *Health Needs Assessment: a practical guide*. London: Health Development Agency; 2005. (HDA functions are now transferred to NICE www.nice.org.uk)

6 Department of Health. *Creating Healthier Communities: a resource pack for local partnerships*. London: Department of Health; 2005.

7 Drinkwater C. *Commissioning Obesity Services: PCTs' services and strategies*. London: NHS Modernisation Agency and NHS Alliance; 2005.

8 Health Development Agency. *Partnerships. Tackling health inequalities. Learning from East and West Midlands*. London: Health Development Agency; 2005.

9 Crisp N. *The Challenges of Commissioning*. Speech made by Sir Nigel Crisp, Chief Executive to the NHS at the NHS Confederation Conference; November 2005.

10 Murphy J. *A Review of the Evidence on Organisational Development for Effective Commissioning in the NHS*. Cambridge: Norfolk, Suffolk and Cambridgeshire Strategic Health Authority; 2005.

11 Powys and Ceredigion Health Promotion. *Programmes – primary health care*. http://healthcare.powys.org.uk/primary.htm

12 Department of Health. *Delivering Choosing Health*. London: Department of Health; 2005.

13 Levy J. *How to Market Better Health. Diabetes. A Dr Foster community health workbook*. London: Dr Foster Ltd; 2005.

14 Ham C, York N, Sutch S et al. Hospital bed utilisation in the NHS. Kaiser Permanente and the US Medicare programme: analysis of routine data. *British Medical Journal*. 2003; **327**: 1257–60.

15 King's Fund. *Predictive Risk Project. Literature review*. London: King's Fund; 2005.

16 Department of Health. *Self Care Support: baseline study of activity and development in self care support in PCTs and local areas*. London: Department of Health; 2005.

17 Department of Health. *Self Care Compendium (Complete)*. London: Department of Health; 2005.

18 Partridge MR and Hill SR on behalf of the 1998 World Asthma Meeting Education and Delivery of Care Working Group. Enhancing care for people with asthma: the role of communication, education, training and self-management. *European Respiratory Journal*. 2000; **16**: 333–48.

19 Kennedy A and Rogers A. Improving self management skills: a whole systems approach. *British Journal of Nursing*. 2001; **10**: 734–7.

4

Getting organised for supporting self care as a general practice team

Ruth Chambers

This chapter describes how you can get organised as a general practice team to design a strategy and implementation plan in relation to supporting self care. The outcome should be a culture whereby supporting self care is integral to all your developments and services, and the GPs and staff promote and support self care as part of their everyday work in effective ways.

Stage 1: getting commitment – developing your vision

Set up your working group or action learning set

A senior team within the practice should form the working group on promoting self care, making the case for a practice strategy and implementation plan – as in the algorithm in Figure 4.1 (adapted from the Faculty of Public Health).[1] Include at least one GP, practice nurse, health care assistant, practice manager, administrative staff member, receptionist and other health professional such as a community pharmacist or a physiotherapist and one or more patient representatives.

Or take up the WiPP training programme and run it as an action learning set (*see* Box 4.1). You will then need someone in your practice team to lead on establishing a self care culture – planning and setting up the action learning set, getting the right people engaged, keeping others motivated, matching learning to people's preferred styles, etc.

Decide whether you will liaise with your PCT to identify a trainer to guide you, or go it alone as a practice team, with your own facilitator as the self care or educational lead. The facilitator of the practice team should be generally experienced in, and work in, the primary care setting. They will usually be the lead for education in a GP team, or a practice manager. Facilitators should be familiar with the principles of self care and contents of the training programme about promoting and supporting self care,[2] so that they can guide their team through the full programme, or extract components of it as suits the team. They should be committed to conveying the importance of good practice in the context of planning and providing primary health care.

Facilitators should advise the team on the amount of preparation and work associated with learning about self care and carrying out agreed actions. They will help to motivate team members to progress smoothly through each stage in their action and learning plans.

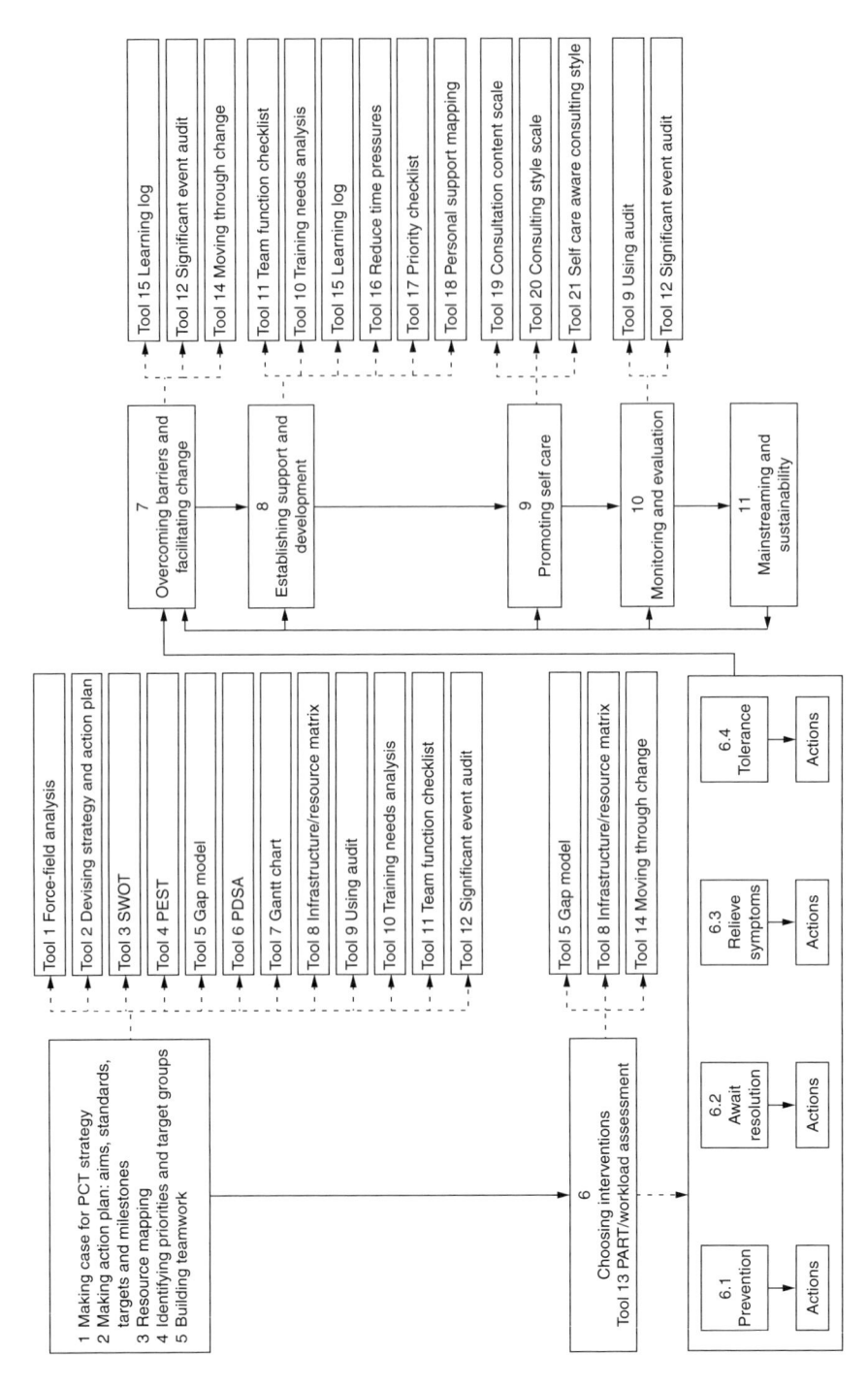

Figure 4.1: Practice team perspective for establishing an integrated resource to support self care.

Getting organised for supporting self care as a general practice team 45

> **Box 4.1:** Using the WiPP multidisciplinary training package in a general practice
>
> Rather than a traditional working group run as part of practice core business, you could use the WiPP training programme to work out your approach as a practice to support self care, and implementing it. The WiPP website has facilitator instructions on running an action learning group and the facilitator's handbook.[2] You can use the electronic versions of the 21 tools (*see* Figure 4.1), or paper versions reproduced in Part 3 of the book, and log your progress.
>
> The WiPP training programme is not prescriptive, as participating practices will be at varying levels of expertise and have different capacity in their evolution of a self care culture. The exact nature of self care support interventions and activities you opt for, will depend on your resources, the nature of your patient population, and your enthusiasm.
>
> Consider the following options:
>
> 1 running an action learning set for a general practice team – around six key members of one practice, or representative leads on self care support from various local practices. Other interested professionals might join in – e.g. community pharmacists, community nurses, allied health professionals. You might meet two- to three-monthly, with time for development and action in between, with shared learning and development under the guidance of a facilitator, not necessarily present at all meetings. We propose a minimum of three facilitated learning and development sessions with intervening associated work being undertaken by individuals and subgroups. Some practices may want to organise more facilitated meetings – the exact arrangements will depend on your preferences and capacity
>
> *or*
>
> 2 a working group to establish an integrated self care support resource within your general practice, with minuted meetings and review of actions to evolve and implement a self care support strategy; with a chair who is a member of the practice team and champion for self care. This is likely to span a minimum of a year.
>
> **The general practice project team**
> Look at the section on teams (pp. 47–8) to confirm your ideas about who can contribute and in what way. Then read through the types of roles and responsibilities various members of the practice team assume in Box 4.2.

The algorithm of Figure 4.1 is similar to that for the PCT approach in Figure 3.1. The only differences between the PCT and practice approaches are in scale and the nature of the patient population. Read through the additional information in the guidance for PCTs in Chapter 3 and generalise to the approach you adopt in your practice.

Look at Tool 1 which explains how to undertake a force-field analysis and consider the positive drivers in deciding to proceed in drawing up and implementing a strategy to support self care across your practice. You can derive many of the positive factors from the evidence for self care support described in Chapter 2. On the opposing side will be the negative factors you should consider before committing to the strategy, and include in your implementation plan with solutions on how to overcome barriers to change.

Use Tool 2 to help you work through the stages of drawing up your strategy and setting priorities. Tool 3 will be useful to analyse strengths, weaknesses, opportunities and threats (SWOT) to establishing a culture of self care in your practice.

Make your aspirations realistic to prevent your vision becoming a mirage.

Drawing up your action plan

Use Tool 4 to consider the political, economic, sociological and technological factors that will influence your practice's action plan. You might prefer to undertake a gap analysis considering where you are now (with unstructured self care initiatives) and where you want to be (Tool 5). Refer back to your vision.

The 'plan, do, study, act' (PDSA) approach of Tool 6 may help you to construct your action plan. Map out a timetable for your prioritised actions – adapting the example Gantt chart in Tool 7 to define your actions and milestones.

Resource mapping

Think about the resources you already have to support self care within your practice, those you will need, and how you might obtain them. Use the infrastructure and resource matrix of Tool 8 to map out your current resources, then plan what extra resources you will need.

You are not building up self care support on your own. Harness the enthusiasm of other general practices, pharmacists and dentists who are supporting self care too. Work with social care, community and voluntary groups and share their resources.

Identify your priorities and target groups

You need to understand your population, know its needs and wants; understand self care and its norms, benchmarks and evidence; understand how to make change. Doing a SWOT analysis and/or audits of your current performance or application of self care (Tool 9) describes your baseline position. This should identify or reaffirm your priorities – the type of self care support and patient groups you will focus on.

Devising an education and training plan for your practice in relation to self care

A culture of promoting effective self care support as a common activity by everyone in the team will only happen if they have the right knowledge and skills, a positive attitude to self care and opportunities to enable it. Your working group or learner set should update your practice training plan to include self care before finalising your strategy and action plan.

1 Just as for any other clinical or practical field, staff in your practice team need to be:
   – competent or qualified to do the job (promote self care) when appointed

or
- correctly trained to an assessed competence before working without supervision.
2 Every staff member should have a personal development plan supported by the practice manager (or other line manager); every GP a personal development plan they review and agree at their annual appraisal.
3 Identify and agree the individual staff member's education and training needs (Tool 10) according to:
   - the requirements of the service for promoting and supporting self care
   - identified individual deficiencies in knowledge, skills or attitudes in relation to supporting self care.
4 Education and training in relation to self care support should be provided in-house (e.g. by a practice lead or PCT trainer) or elsewhere, and the time allowed to do this.

If you are encouraging individual staff to take on responsibilities outside their traditional role in supporting patients' self care you must ensure that the tasks are:

- within their personal skills and competence
- carried out after an enhancement of their knowledge or skills
- not compromising their existing duties
- best carried out by them and not by others with different roles or skills
- organised so that they are able to be personally accountable for their actions.

Building your team

Your practice team will implement your self care support strategy. So try out Tool 11 to check how well your team is functioning, and/or undertake a significant event audit as in Tool 12.

Good communication is essential for good teamwork.[3–5] You need:

- regular staff meetings which everyone endeavours to attend
- a failsafe system for passing on important messages
- ways to share news so that everyone is promptly notified of changes
- a culture where team members can speak openly without fear of being judged or reprimanded
- opportunities for quieter members of the team to contribute
- to give and receive feedback on how roles in the team are working out
- to praise others for their achievements
- opportunities for team members to point out problems and suggest improvements
- everyone to be part of, and own, the decision making.

Teams which encourage participation are more likely to achieve a patient-centred service, to work together as a team and be more efficient.[3,4] Look at the range of roles and responsibilities of a typical team in Box 4.2. If you are unaware of Belbin's description of team roles, you can read about that elsewhere.[6]

Box 4.2: Forming a coherent primary care team for your self care support initiative: who does what

The practice manager

- Understands the characteristics of effective teams and how to encourage their development
- Obtains facts and figures about team members' learning needs in relation to self care
- Involves all team members and communicates regularly with them
- Encourages attached staff and independent contractors to join in the practice action plan, promoting and supporting self care
- Arranges regular learning and review meetings with all staff and encourages everyone to be involved
- Identifies necessary resources for supporting self care
- Oversees audit and monitoring of the self care support initiative

The GP

- Leads on writing the strategy and implementation plan for the practice team to promote self care
- Encourages multiprofessional working and values individual members' contributions
- Joins in multiprofessional learning and training with the team in relation to consultation techniques for supporting self care
- Provides adequate resources for staff to have sufficient opportunities for learning development

The practice nurse

- Is flexible about fitting in with new requirements for different ways of working in relation to supporting self care
- Contributes to teaching patients and colleagues about self care
- Actively seeks out, and participates in, learning and training in relation to self care support
- Supervises the health care assistant who promotes self care to patients

The receptionist and health care assistant

- Attends project and staff meetings
- Joins in multiprofessional learning and training with other team members
- Becomes familiar with self care literature and distributes this to patients
- Helps the practice manager obtain data for the evaluation of the self care support initiative
- Passes on information to colleagues who are unable to attend a meeting

The patient and/or carer representative

- Attends self care planning meetings
- Contributes her/his own ideas and views and passes on suggestions and comments from other patients and/or patients' group

- Participates in writing and testing of patient information systems
- Advises on patient/consumer perspectives

Others, e.g. health visitor, midwife, community pharmacist, physiotherapist, community psychiatric nurse, specialist nurse

- Joins the practice team to contribute to the self care support initiative as an expert in his/her own specialty
- Agrees his/her own role and responsibility within the initiative

Understand what motivates your team in order to achieve the best results from them. It is said that performance = ability × motivation.[7]

Take team development seriously, following tried and tested approaches.[8] Base it on the core business of the practice such as ensuring clinical governance, so that you tie your self care support initiative into other developments within the practice.[9] If most team members have similar learning needs such as in relation to self care aware consultation skills, then consider holding a workshop on the topic in the practice or at an away day, to encourage team building too.[10] Include patient representatives in your development team too – they can accelerate change and help with finding solutions to overcome barriers to progress in implementing the self care support strategy – *see* Chapters 5 and 7 for more on working with patients.[11]

Stage 2: choosing one or two conditions to focus your self care support initiative on

The interventions you select will depend on your practice priorities and target groups. Tool 13 will be key to action planning as it assesses the clinical and organisational workload generated by a variety of example health conditions. Then consider what you and patients can do in respect of those conditions in relation to:

P: **P**reventing the condition developing
A: **A**waiting resolution of the symptoms
R: using self care skills for **R**elief of symptoms
T: learning to **T**olerate symptoms that do not resolve or cannot be reasonably alleviated.

Your PCT may be able to support your efforts with parallel community initiatives.

Try out on a patient pathway to self care

Chapters 10 to 13 illustrate four different patient pathways in relation to conditions about which patients commonly consult their GP or triage nurse, and for which there are plenty of self care options: sore throat, back pain, asthma and cough and colds.

Work through one or more of our example patient scenarios and fictional practice team action planning in Chapters 10 to 13, as a practice team. You can:

- read through a patient story and the discussions and actions the fictional practice team take in responding to the patient story to optimise self care. Then consider how it applies to your practice

or

- substitute your own patient story – a recent consultation maybe – and get ready to work through the same stages as the fictional team to get your own action plan and outcomes.

The learning issues that could result from such a team discussion appear throughout the sequence of the scenario. What you discuss and learn depends on members of your group, their situations, their interests, your resources, and the skills of your facilitator or lead. Examples of advice and guidance you might relay to patients are given in each chapter. Alternatively, you can direct them to the associated algorithm from NHS Direct.[12]

Choose one of the four conditions we have illustrated or use your own topic, and research the various self care support options or look at more examples on the WiPP website.[2] To decide your priority conditions, identify the frequency with which patients are consulting for specific conditions in your practice or group of practices, using the workload assessment tool (*see* Tool 13). After that, focus your initial activity for supporting self care for people with long term conditions whom you identify as being frequent consulters at your practice, or who have had several emergency admissions in the last 12 months. Tool 3 (SWOT analysis) or Tool 5 (gap analysis) might help you select which interventions will be a priority for your practice. Read through Chapter 2 for more ideas on self care support initiatives that others have tried, that you could adapt. Consider the resource implications of your chosen interventions using Tool 8.

Stage 3: keeping going

Look back at Figure 4.1 which maps your route to establishing a self care culture across your practice with self care routinely promoted effectively.

Everyone in your practice team should be clear about practice goals, their roles and responsibilities, the timetabled programmes for improvements, and standards required.

Overcoming barriers and facilitating change

The most commonly perceived barriers to supporting self care initially in the *Joining Up Self Care* initiative were described in Box 3.5 (*see* p. 40).

Encourage team members to keep a learning log during their everyday practice, as in Tool 15, or to undertake a significant event audit relating to trying to promote self care – and succeeding or failing (*see* Tool 12). Consider what worked well, and what got in the way, using Tools 12 and 14 or any other Tools. Then find solutions to overcome barriers and move towards supporting self care as part of everyday practice.

Establishing support and development

Concentrate on meeting team members' learning needs (*see* Tool 10), sustaining good teamworking (*see* Tool 11), encouraging reflection on performance and learning from experience (*see* Tool 15). Rethink the way that you book consultations and that patients access services so that there is time to promote self care during consultations (*see* Tool 16). Check everyone has self care as a priority for learning and service development, using Tool 17.

Supporting self care

You need to encourage good patient-centred consultation techniques across the practice team. Advocate Tools 19 and 20 to check out everyone's consultation skills and styles. You could use Tool 21 as a core component of a workshop on self care aware consultation techniques for an in-house workshop. Complete our aide mémoire (the last stage of Tool 21) as a progress report to trigger reflection on improving your approach (*see* Box 4.3).

Box 4.3: Complete your aide mémoire recording your progress in actioning self care support and considering what else you can do to be more effective

1 What have you tried already?
2 How long have you tried this for?
3 What were you trying to achieve by doing this?
4 Has it worked and how?
5 Have you stopped doing what you tried and why?
6 What could you do next time?

Remember that promoting self care will be tough. Anything new that requires patients to make significant changes will be difficult and, to your team already working under pressure, may seem an overwhelming task. Encourage your workforce and health professional community to look after themselves too. Tool 18 is a good start, for individuals to map out the types and extent of support in their own lives, and see which sources of support can be boosted.

Stage 4: monitoring and evaluation

Evaluation is an essential component of any programme or service. Incorporate it into your action plan from the beginning, matched to your vision and aims. Keep it as simple as possible and do not waste resources on unnecessarily bureaucratic evaluation. Use Tools 9 and 12 to undertake audits of self care outputs and activities being generated by your self care support strategy and its implementation. Look at Chapter 9 for more on evaluation.

Mainstreaming and sustaining a self care culture in your practice

You will have generated a co-ordinated series of activities and developments leading to the promotion of self care among patients with the priority health condition(s) you have selected. Re-assess your priorities and resource needs as you gather data evaluating your progress to date. You will be moving in a circular fashion to re-examine barriers to progress and facilitate further change (*see* Figure 4.1).

References

1 Swanton K. *A Toolkit for Developing a Local Strategy to Tackle Overweight and Obesity in Adults and Children*. London: Faculty of Public Health; 2005.
2 www.wipp.nhs.uk
3 Poulton B and West M. The determinants of effectiveness in primary health care teams. *Journal of Interprofessional Care*. 1999; **13:** 7–18.
4 Hart E and Fletcher J. Learning how to change: a selective analysis of literature and experience of how teams learn and organisations change. *Journal of Interprofessional Care*. 1999; **13:** 53–63.
5 McDerment L. *Stress Care*. Surrey: Social Care Association (Education); 1988.
6 Belbin RM. *Management Teams, why they Succeed or Fail*. London: Heinemann; 1991.
7 Dibben C. Topics on motivating a team. *BMJ Careers*. 2005; **23 April:** 167.
8 McMillan R and Kelly D. A project of Team Involvement in Development and Learning (TIDAL). *Education for Primary Care*. 2005; **16:** 175–83.
9 Thomas M. Team learning: understanding clinical governance. *Work Based Learning in Primary Care*. 2004; **2:** 277–9.
10 Kennedy A, Gask L and Rogers A. Training professionals to engage with and promote self-management. *Health Education Research*. 2005; **20:** 567–78.
11 Clinical Governance Support Team. *Patients Accelerating Change. Working in Partnership with Patients. Resource Pack*. Leicester: Clinical Governance Support Team and Picker Institute Europe; 2005.
12 NHS Direct. www.nhsdirect.nhs.uk

5

Getting organised for supporting self care as an individual professional in the general practice team

Ruth Chambers

This chapter shows you how you can best promote and support self care as a health professional as part of your everyday work, linking in with others in your practice team.

GPs and other health professionals working in primary care share similar core competencies: primary care management, person-centred care, specific problem solving skills, comprehensive approach, community orientation and holistic modelling which include the psychosocial and cultural dimensions of a person's life.[1]

The six competencies shown in Figure 5.1 are rooted in:

- the attitudes of health professionals and patients
- the evidence base or science of medical management and treatment
- the context of the primary care setting and the person.[2,3]

As patients become better informed, the GP, nurse, allied health professional (AHP), pharmacist or other health professional should encourage patients to use their expertise in taking care of their own illnesses and in changing to more healthy behaviour. The general practice team can build their relationship with the patient, deal with health problems in their physical, psychological, social, cultural and existential dimensions, and reinforce consistent health messages.

How the health care practitioner can enable patients to self care

According to patients, health care professionals can enable self care by:

- establishing effective two-way communication between health care professional and patient
- building a good relationship between practitioner and patient: treating patients holistically and establishing trust
- providing patients with information on their disease and signposting other local resources
- developing self care plans for individual patients
- sharing decision making with patients about their management and care
- using motivational techniques with patients
- signposting or recommending over-the-counter medicines

- encouraging patients to access reliable health information[4]
- referring patients to self care skills training
- directing patients to self care support networks in the community.

Developing and sustaining an effective communication style

Key aspects of effective communication include rapport, empathy, listening, questioning, being non-judgemental, being consistent and using the same type of language as that of the patient (*see* Box 5.1). Some patients like to know detailed medical terms, in part so that they can undertake their own research. You should understand cultural diversity, since diseases are viewed differently by various groups of patients, and those differences can have an impact on individuals' motivation to self care. Be flexible, i.e. adapt your own style according to the needs of the individual patient. Communication needs to be uniformly good – between all types of health professionals, and by an individual health professional whether or not they are having a pressured day or are on 'top' form.

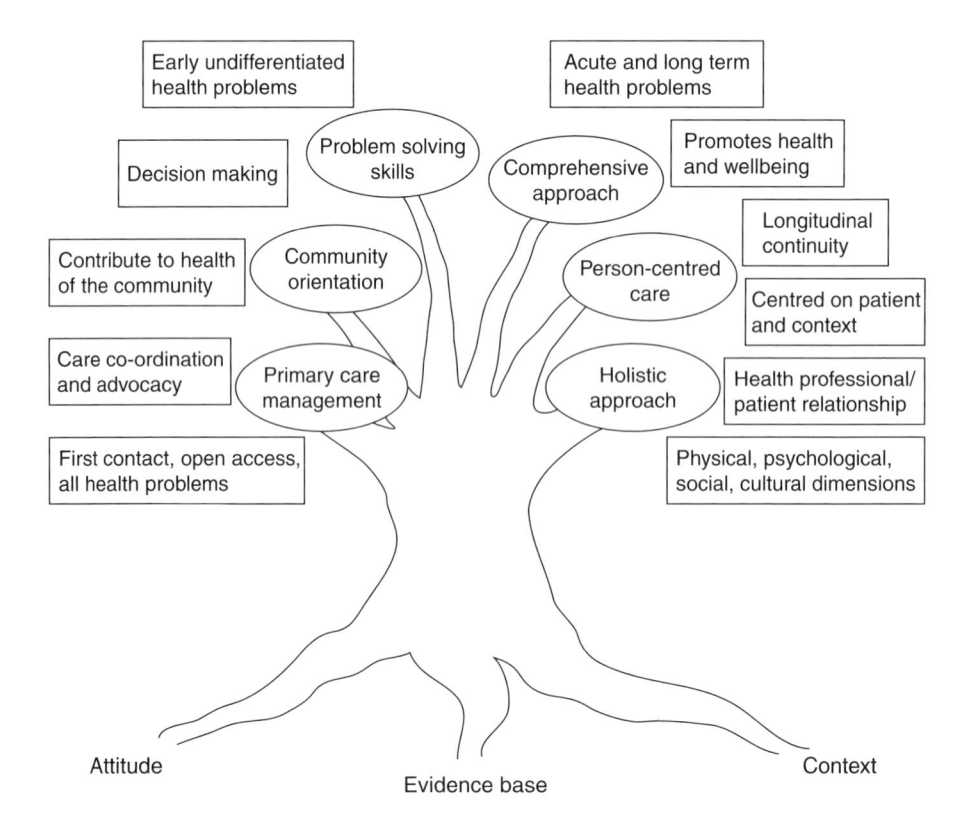

Figure 5.1: The interrelation of core competencies of primary health care professionals, implementation areas and background features of general practice (adapted from Grueninger[3]).

> Box 5.1: What patients perceive as effective communication by health
> professionals
> - Using language that is 'down-to-earth', non-clinical
> - Talking openly and frankly about the condition
> - Using humour
> - Being informal and using positive expression
> - Being friendly and caring[4]

Use Tool 19 to assess your consultation skills and style, to check that you are taking up opportunities to promote self care to patients and are providing them with a wide choice of self care support. Or try Tool 20 to ensure that you are being as patient centred as you think you are in your everyday consultations with patients.

Limited consultation time emphasises the importance of effective communication. Areas to include are: listening, questioning (relevant to understanding motivational issues and treating the patient holistically), building rapport, use of appropriate language, and providing consistent communication. You need to be able to communicate across cultural boundaries to engage with patients of all backgrounds.

Look at the content of Figure 5.2. Have good eye contact at the beginning of the consultation and at reasonable intervals throughout; ask about the patient's perceptions and feelings; use active listening to clarify what patients are concerned about, and avoid interrupting the patient before they have finished giving you the essentials. Knowing about the signs indicating someone's background mental state helps you to understand not just what is said but the feelings behind the words.

The meaning of language

Most of the time you understand what people say, but sometimes your 'wires get crossed'.[5] Some examples of poor language skills are:

- *action meanings*: people often use action statements when they do not like to ask directly for things. Saying 'It's very fresh in here with the window open' can be a request for the window to be shut, and the speaker will be quite offended if you reply 'Yes, it's nice to have fresh air coming in'
- *taking things literally*: the answer to 'Have you seen that file I put down?' is not 'Yes' but 'It's over there on the table'
- *connotative meanings*: these can suggest emotions but express what is said and what is meant differently. Many people remember their full name being used when someone was telling them off. People who use metaphors implying that the workplace is a war zone may be expressing their inner feelings about it being a battlefield
- *using jargon*: the use of jargon can sometimes be an unconscious attempt to prevent communication and understanding – after all if you do not understand what I am talking about you cannot possibly do my job! More often, it is the failure to use feedback (or lack of it) to modify what is being said to the level of understanding of the listener.

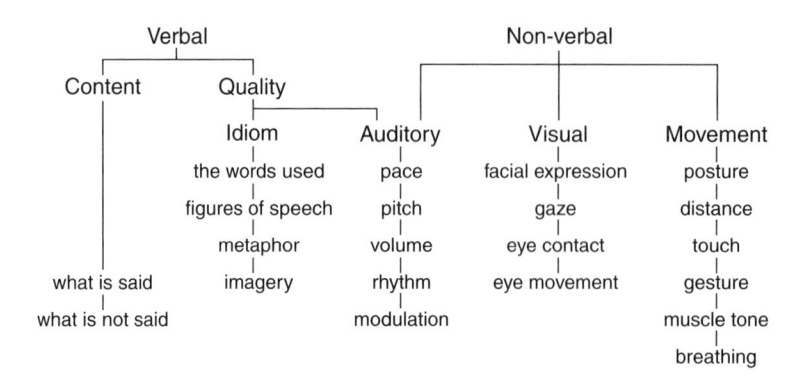

```
                    Verbal                              Non-verbal
          ┌───────────┴──────────┐           ┌──────────────┼──────────────┐
       Content                Quality
          │           ┌──────────┼──────────┐
          │         Idiom     Auditory      │          Visual           Movement
          │           │           │                       │                │
          │    the words used    pace              facial expression    posture
          │           │           │                       │                │
          │    figures of speech pitch                   gaze           distance
          │           │           │                       │                │
          │       metaphor     volume                eye contact         touch
          │           │           │                       │                │
     what is said  imagery     rhythm               eye movement        gesture
          │                       │                                        │
     what is not said          modulation                              muscle tone
                                                                           │
                                                                        breathing
```

Figure 5.2: Signs of the mental state in communication. Note that cultural factors may influence what is happening, e.g. the amount of eye contact, gesture or touch.

Building a positive relationship and developing trust

Two important aspects of the patient/health care professional relationship are: being treated holistically as a whole person and developing trust (*see* Box 5.2).

Treating the patient holistically means evaluating all the factors that can influence a patient's behaviour, including their overall health status, mental wellbeing (such as mood and self-esteem) and their personal circumstances. Undertake an evaluation of all of a patient's health conditions when deciding with them on their treatment. Look at all the factors likely to impact on their ability to self care (including their mood), your style of communication, and other health options such as complementary medicine. Use goal setting (e.g. as part of a self care plan), positive feedback and positive thinking approaches to build up their confidence and self-efficacy.

Box 5.2: Patients' perspectives as to how health professionals can enhance self care by building good relationships

Treat the patient holistically

- Treat the patient as a whole person not just a single condition
- Evaluate all the factors that might impact on self care such as mental wellbeing, other health conditions and personal circumstances
- Consider complementary therapies if appropriate

Trust

- Build on continuity of your relationship and care with the patient
- Honesty:
  - be open about not knowing everything
  - don't be frightened to tell hard truths e.g. the need to change diet or exercise – this encourages self responsibility

Working as a partnership

- Your consultation should be a two-way discussion

Getting organised for supporting self care as an individual professional

Building trust is closely linked to effective health professional–patient communication. Trust should be a central focus in relationship building with patients and building rapport. Building trust includes: good communication skills (e.g. consistency of communication), honesty (e.g. being honest about uncertainties of the condition and admitting to not knowing everything) and practical elements such as confidentiality. See how a patient describes the need for trust in Box 5.3 and what people value in Box 5.4.

> **Box 5.3:** A patient describing the need to build a trusting relationship with their family doctor
>
> 'Trust is actually vital, it's really important, I think for me. In my doctor's surgery there are certain doctors I do trust but there are others I would not see. It's the way they talk to me, it's showing respect. They actually listen to what I have to say. It's also for them to realise that even though you are a doctor, it's like every profession, you don't know everything, there's always something new that you need to learn. With my doctor the thing that I like about him is that he constantly updates his knowledge ... I'm always passing information to him, he says "that's wonderful I didn't know about that."'

You can encourage people to trust you if you:
- do what you say you will do and do not make promises you can't or won't keep
- listen to people carefully and tell them what you think they are saying. People trust others whom they believe understand them
- understand what matters to people. People trust those who are looking out for their best interests.

> **Box 5.4:** Relationships with health professionals in primary care are mostly good
>
> A survey of 117 000 patients by the Healthcare Commission gave broadly positive impressions of their experiences of primary care services, including care by doctors and dentists.[6] Patients want fast access to good care. They want to have a say in their care and be enabled to help themselves. Seventy-six per cent of patients reported that they definitely had confidence and trust in the doctor whom they saw; 75% were confident in their dentist; 92% of people said the doctor whom they saw always treated them with dignity and respect, but 18% felt they had not been given enough information about potential side-effects by their GP. Sixty-nine per cent said they were involved as much as they wanted to be by GPs in decisions about their care and treatment; 70% said their dentist involved them enough.

Patients want to see the same person over several visits. Otherwise, seeing different individuals on various occasions can mean that patients have to repeat the same information and may receive conflicting advice.

Providing reliable information

You need to focus on providing disease information that is tailored to the individual patient, encompassing both detailed background on their condition as well as self care skills (e.g. self-monitoring and managing diet). Highlight other sources of information, such as local self care support networks, free exercise programmes, especially tailored information for individual cultures/nationalities, such as local diet sheets (e.g. for West/East African, Asian nationalities etc). Signpost them to reliable resources on the internet too (*see* 'Promoting effective use of health information by patients', p. 66).

Practice nurses and nurse practitioners, diabetes specialist nurses and other specialist nurses, in particular, provide useful, in-depth, information on a patient's disease as well as giving practical advice on self care in a style to which patients respond well (e.g. in an interactive way). Patients value health professionals taking the time to provide detailed information that is relevant to them, and not taking for granted what they may or may not already understand about their condition.

Emphasise the following elements of disease education with individual patients: basic knowledge of their disease, individual risk factors, long term implications of their disease, and the consequences of not self caring. Guide them about the types of questions to ask when pursuing further knowledge of the disease, for example, with hospital specialists.

Encouraging patients' self care skills

If you are able to establish effective patient-centred communication then you are more likely to encourage and support patients in taking decisions and in their self care actions to take optimal care of their health condition outside of health service settings.[7] The skills that you should use as part of the patient-centred approach are described in Box 5.5.

Box 5.5:   The patient-centred approach to promote and support self care

1 *Exploring the disease and illness experience*:
   – what are they worried or unhappy about?
   – personal and psychological impact of disease
   – how to recognise and treat flare-ups immediately
   – recognise situations when help is needed

2 *The whole person – understanding their role and position in life*:
   – how do treatment regimes fit in with their working and personal lives?
   – can they work during a flare-up?
   – any problems in self treatment?

3 *Finding common ground between them and you*:
   - what decisions (shared decision making) have to be made about: lifestyle, drug treatment, living with side-effects, surgery, surveillance, quality of disease management versus medical efficacy?
   - make entries in patient held records together: test results, everyday maintenance treatment, how to recognise symptoms of flare-ups and treatment regime for self care of flare-ups.
4 *Prevention and health promotion*:
   - starting treatment fast
   - removing unnecessary stresses from life
   - importance of routine medication
   - how to access others e.g. dietitian
5 *Enhancing the patient–professional relationship*:
   - acknowledge areas of uncertainties
   - allow patients to take responsibility for self care
   - write down an overall self care plan including a personal treatment plan
   - make follow-up appointments on request
   - recognise the legitimacy of patients' non-medical approaches to care
6 *Being realistic, ensure understanding*:
   - making sure patients understand and are happy with joint management and decisions
   - not dumping all uncertainties on patients[7]

The development of self care support programmes requires joint decision making between the patient and health professional, which in turn helps to promote self care – as in Box 5.6. Currently, self care plans appear to focus mainly on treatment issues (e.g. self administration of medication for asthma patients). Self care training should cover: medical issues, emotional and psychological issues, how to work with various health care professionals providing care for their disease, and making lifestyle changes. Cognitive techniques and support from other patients in self care support networks and peer-to-peer groups are options that are particularly useful for patients with mental health problems. Cognitive behavioural therapy (CBT) skills can be applied in all consultations. CBT encourages patient involvement, autonomy and increased concordance. Health professionals and patients work together to understand ongoing problems. This technique could be included in self care plans, to encourage joint decision making, tailored to the individual.

Box 5.6: A practice nurse encourages self care with a self care plan for asthma

'With my asthma patients what I do is I give them an action plan. I try to encourage them to recognise what brings the asthma on and be able to avoid it when they can, and once they can do that it means they can stop and start their

> treatments at the right time ... an action plan that they can follow in terms of adding in and taking out medication ... about when to contact their doctor, how to avoid an emergency ... there's no point in taking an inhaler all year round ... it's about teaching them to self-monitor ... They also get a peak flow meter ... if they feel any deterioration they just blow into the little machine and it gives them an idea of what's happening and what they might be able to do.'[4]

In one study, cognitive behavioural-based self help mental health care facilitated by practice nurses was as effective as ordinary care, with similar costs; patients participating were more satisfied with facilitated self help too.[8]

You could use Tool 21 to review the various stages you go through in a typical consultation with a patient, and check that you are challenging, guiding, suggesting, encouraging, stimulating and generally optimising the promotion of self care. Or guide patients to the 'Self care for people' training course (*see* Box 5.7).

> **Box 5.7:** 'Self Care for People' training course[9]
>
> This self care skills training course has volunteer trainers to co-lead the courses. It should help people to:
>
> - be motivated and empowered to develop self care behaviours
> - know where to gain access to further information and services
> - take responsibility for their own and/or other people's health
> - make informed decisions about accessing available services.

Sharing decision making

As a health professional, you should respect the values and beliefs of patients and not try to impose your own attitudes upon them. The feelings of loss of control, vulnerability and isolation that accompany illness leave people open to manipulative behaviour by their carers and health workers. A potential imbalance of power is created by your superior knowledge as the provider of services. Shared decision making is the middle ground between informed choice, where decisions are left entirely to the patient, and traditional, paternalistic medical decision making. It involves two-way information giving (medical and personal) between the clinician and patient concerning all options available, with the final decision being made jointly with both parties in total agreement.[9] To share information and relate well requires you to consider how you interact with a patient in respect of:

- *partnership*: help for someone with a problem through partnership between that person and professionals
- *empowerment*: help for those with problems to find the best ways of helping themselves
- *judgement*: beware of judgement – the person with the problem is the only one who really understands their experience and problem

- *values*: people's values and priorities change with time; they may be quite different from your values, but no less valid
- *autonomy*: autonomy should be a fundamental right of everyone. Illness, disability, low income, unemployment and other forms of social exclusion mean a loss of some aspects of autonomy in society
- *listening*: active non-judgemental listening is core to helping people, and crucial to gain an understanding of people with problems
- *shared decision making*: people with ongoing problems need to be able to take their own decisions about the care of their clinical condition, based on expert information communicated to them by professionals. Patients do value shared decision making, but not as much as other key attributes of consultations such as having a doctor who listens, and being provided with easily understood information.[10] Shared decision making leads into concordance, which should be the goal of all shared decision making encounters between health professional and patient[11]
- *concordance*: a negotiated agreement on the management of a clinical problem between the person with the problem and the professional allows the patient to take an informed decision on the degree of risk or suffering that they themselves wish to take on.[12] In contrast 'compliance' with treatment, lifestyle or other changes, implies that the patient follows instructions from professionals to a greater or lesser degree. *See* Box 5.8 for more on this.

Box 5.8: Concordance is the right approach to encourage patient involvement and their self care

'Concordance is fundamentally different from either compliance or adherence ... in that it focuses on the consultation process rather than on a specific patient behaviour, and it has an underlying ethos of a shared approach to decision making rather than paternalism.'[13]

Concordance has four elements:[14]

1 *patients have enough knowledge to participate as partners*:
   - they have access to information about their condition, treatment options available and risks and benefits of different options relative to their own situation
   - education empowers patients to take care of their own health
   - patients feel confident in asking questions and engaging in discussion about medicines

2 *consultations involve patients as partners*:
   - patients can talk about taking medicines
   - professionals explain the agreed treatment fully
   - patients are as involved as they want to be in treatment decisions
   - patients and health professionals reach a joint understanding of the decision
   - a patient's ability to follow treatment is checked

3 *patients are supported in taking medicines*:
 - medication is reviewed regularly with patients
 - all opportunities used to discuss treatment are taken
 - practical difficulties in taking treatment are discussed
 - information about patients is effectively shared between professionals
4 *health professionals are prepared for partnership*:
 - health professionals are equipped with the necessary skills to engage patients
 - health professionals regard investment of time in reaching an informed agreement as important.

Involving patients in making treatment decisions poses concerns for their health professionals. These include the extra time needed and difficulties in eliciting patients' preferences, exacerbated by limited appropriate information to support patient involvement. Health professionals may not have the appropriate competencies (*see* p. 70) such as ability to communicate risk effectively or accept patient preferences that are different from their own or evidence based guidelines. Some clinicians prefer to retain the imbalance of power between themselves and their patients; some patients may be reluctant to express their preferences if they perceive their doctor or nurse as being more powerful and knowledgeable.[15,16]

Certain catchphrases and open questions have been advocated as being useful for involving patients in decision making. Examples are given in Box 5.9.

Box 5.9: 'Catchphrases' and open questions that health professionals might use to involve patients in decision making

Exploring patient expectations
'What do you want to get out of our appointment today?'
'What would you like to see happen here?'

Exploring patient ideas
'What are your thoughts as to what is going on here?'
'Do you have any ideas as to what this might be?'

Exploring patient concerns
'Is there anything else you would like to know about?'
'Is there anything in particular that worries you?'
'Have you had any bad experiences with this kind of thing in the past?'

Identifying options
'Have you thought about any alternatives?'
'There are several options here that we could try'

Determining patient preferences for information
'What do you know about it?'
'Would you like to know more?'
'What do you want to know about it?'

'How would you like this information? Some people like to read things, others prefer pictures or diagrams, while other people like numbers . . .'

Determining a patient's preference for their role in decision making
'How would you feel if we both thought through the various options together?'
'Do you want to be more involved in our decisions here?'[17]

There are a variety of consultation models that you might consider and adapt in supporting self care. Most start with establishing rapport with the patient, exploring their reasons for the consultation, being aware of the doctor's agenda, reaching a shared understanding and formulating an action plan together.

Enhancing patients' motivation to self care

Personal motivation is one of the main characteristics of the patient that determines the level of self care they attain. Motivation is influenced by the individual patient's personality type, age, level of education, and social class. Motivation is also affected by mental wellbeing, knowledge about their disease, type of support from others and their cultural background. Motivation can either be intrinsic or extrinsic. Intrinsic motivation might be about someone enjoying learning about self care and practising it, for their own sake; feeling confident that they have the tools to self care. Extrinsic motivation might be either in the form of a 'carrot or a stick', rewards or adverse events.

The main approaches appear to be:

- treating the patient holistically, which involves exploring all current reasons for their low motivation to self care (e.g. mood, social circumstances)
- building confidence and 'self-efficacy' by setting achievable goals and then providing positive feedback and encouragement (see Box 5.10)
- being flexible in approach: negotiating with patients and adopting a different style in order to achieve the desired outcome
- providing knowledge of the disease (see p. 66)
- developing a range of self care support options.[4]

Box 5.10: Tips on boosting patients' motivation to self care

'Some people have poor motivation because they have never achieved . . . so they don't feel in control so it's about showing them the small things that they can achieve . . . so that they can have that self-efficacy.'[4] (GP)

'We are trying to initiate self care . . . Patients need to learn about their illnesses and how to monitor them, as well as where to go for more education. We are encouraging them to take more responsibility.'[18] (GP prize winner of enterprise award)

To motivate patients, you need to use techniques to build patients' self confidence and self-efficacy which involve goal setting and providing positive feedback and encouragement. You could also use approaches such as re-framing (changing negatives into positives) and positive self-talk to help motivate those with a 'negative outlook'. These sort of approaches and techniques for listening and questioning are described in neuro-linguistic programming (NLP), motivational interviewing, and social cognitive theory.[19,20]

Heron's six categories of intervention describe the different help-giving approaches that you can adopt when face-to-face with an individual patient.[21] The first three represent energy flowing from the health professional, who is actively intervening to alter the patient's thinking or behaviour. In the other three categories, the health professional is playing a less active role, attempting to induce the patient to think or behave differently:

1 *prescriptive*: giving advice, being critical, making suggestions and generally attempting to direct the behaviour of the individual
2 *informative*: instructing, informing and generally imparting factual information to the individual
3 *confronting*: being challenging or giving direct feedback to a patient to challenge their attitudes, beliefs or behaviours, while assuming a supportive manner
4 *cathartic*: helping someone to express their feelings and emotions to enable them to gain new insights into their condition
5 *catalytic*: drawing the other person out through the use of open questions, reflection and empathy, encouraging them in learning more about themselves and problem solving
6 *supportive*: approving, confirming or validating someone's experience, qualities, attitudes or actions, in a genuine way.

Thinking of the pros and cons of the various options open to a person and visualising what that means in real life is a great way to motivate people – as in Box 5.11.

Box 5.11: Motivational advice from a health column in a local newspaper

Q: I desperately want to lose weight and have taken out gym membership but never been to use the facilities. Please help me get motivated.

A: Make a list of the pro and cons for the current situation you're in. So on the plus side, you have more time at home, and are not risking pulling a muscle at the gym. On the minus side, you're wasting the money you paid to join the gym, you're overweight and you're unfit. Next, make a list of the pros and cons if you start going regularly to the gym. On the plus side, you'll get fit, meet new friends, regain your self-esteem, take pride in your appearance. On the minus side – difficult to think of anything. Lastly, work out what is stopping you going to the gym when there are self-obviously so many pluses to be had. Think out how you will do it, and make a personal action plan.[22]

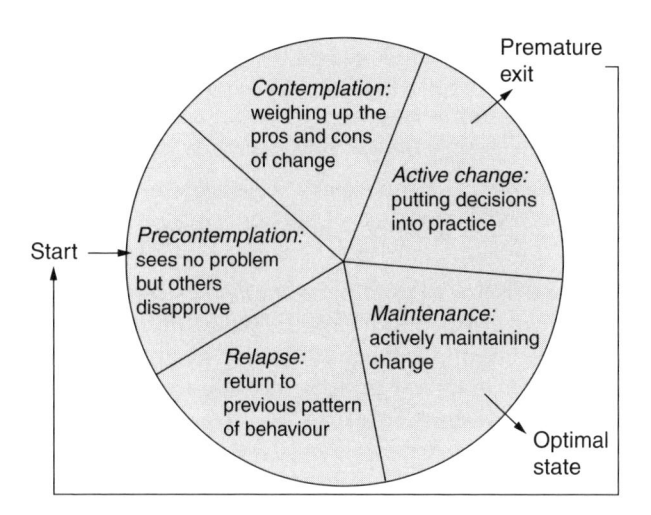

Figure 5.3: Cycle of change.

Helping people change

The model in Figure 5.3 describes the stages in the cycle of change through which an individual moves, and how they must be motivated to change.[23] It was initially developed for smoking cessation, then used for many other health behaviour programmes. Behaviour change is not a linear movement through these stages though. It can be progressive, regressive, spiralling or static; people may skip one or more stages or stick in one for a long time.

It is essential to choose an appropriate time to motivate a person to change, such as from risky habits to a healthy lifestyle. Hopefully, individuals pass through the stage of contemplation and onto the stage of taking action for themselves. You should set realistic targets for that change that are achievable so as not to demotivate the person or allow them an escape route ('I knew I couldn't do it'). It can be difficult to assess what stage someone is in – especially if the health professional is pressed for time. You can make assumptions and mistakenly rate someone as being ready to change, so the more you can involve the other person in rating where they are themselves, the better.

Everyone likes to get feedback and encouragement about how they are doing. Do not just leave it until an annual health check, give the patient praise when and where it is due at any time.

Signposting or recommending over-the-counter (OTC) medicines

Signpost people to the various range of treatments they can buy themselves without a prescription. Use an evidence based resource to make your recommendations.[24] *See* Chapter 6 for more on this. Increased switching from prescription only medicines (POM) to pharmacy medicines (P) has meant that the public can self treat more conditions, e.g. emergency contraception as described in Box 5.12.[25] It has implications for training of patients, doctors and nurses about what is possible, and pharmacists about their increased role.[26] There is more to be done in educating the public – one study found that an estimated 8% of adult attendances at an accident and emergency department could have been managed by a community pharmacist.[27]

> **Box 5.12:** Greater use of pharmacies to access emergency contraception
>
> Emergency contraception became available without a prescription from community pharmacies in 2001. The percentage of women obtaining emergency contraceptive pills from a pharmacy has increased markedly from 27% in 2003–2004 to 50% in 2004–2005. Over the same time period, the proportions of women getting the 'morning after pill' from a GP or practice nurse fell to 33%, from a walk-in centre or minor-injuries unit fell to 3%, and from a family planning clinic remained stable at 11%.[25]
>
> OTC medicines bring both benefits and risks. Benefits include enabling people to take more responsibility for their own health or that of their dependants with rapid and convenient access to treatments and use health professional capacity more efficiently. Potential risks include adverse effects (*see* Box 5.17, p. 76) and possible misuse of certain medicines.[28]

Promoting effective use of health information by patients

Disease information should be specific to the needs of the individual (i.e. the right information for the right stage of the condition and the nature of the person). Health care professionals should be familiar with the variety of local self care support networks and peer-to-peer support groups that are available as sources of disease education. Patients want qualitative information – not just the facts and figures. They want to know what it is like to live with a particular condition, not just the treatment options. They want to know how their condition will affect their ability to work, their usual activities, their family relationships, and their sex life.

At present, there is an enormous amount of information about health and medicines available from many different sources but it is not always easy for patients to access.[29,30] Nor is it always clear how reliable, authoritative or up-to-date such sources of information are. Information about medicines and disease states, and suggestions for self care, are provided:

- in doctors' surgery waiting rooms, pharmacies, hospitals and clinics
- by professional bodies
- by health charities and patient support groups
- in libraries
- via the internet
- via the media.

We provide patients with information to:

- help them understand what is wrong
- gain a realistic idea of their prognosis
- make the most of consultations

- understand the process and likely outcomes of possible tests and treatments
- assist in self care
- provide reassurance and help to cope
- help others understand
- legitimise help seeking and concerns
- identify further information and self care support networks and groups
- identify the 'best' health care providers.[31]

Information about risks and benefits of medicines, safe use of medicines and what actions people can take for themselves may not be explicit. Information may not be phrased in language or presented visually in ways that the majority of patients easily comprehend. Information leaflets or other media do not necessarily cater for non-English speakers or people from different cultures.

A good-quality publication about treatment choices will:

- have explicit aims and achieve them
- be relevant to consumers
- make date and sources of information explicit
- be balanced and unbiased
- refer to areas of uncertainty
- describe how treatment works – its benefits, the risks and what would happen without treatment
- describe effects of treatment choices on overall quality of life
- make it clear about range of treatment choices
- provide support for shared decision making
- list additional sources of information.[32]

You can use the DISCERN instrument to determine whether your patient literature fulfils the quality criteria listed above.[32]

When judging the impact of patient literature, consider the:

- writing style
- typeface
- design and layout
- headings
- use of colour
- use of symbols.[29]

See Box 5.13 for a good example.

Box 5.13: A brilliant example of literature for the general public

The Haynes Owners Workshop Manual is a cleverly produced practical guide to healthy living and weight loss for men. It is modelled on the Haynes' manuals for various makes of car, and entitled *HGV Man – reducing all large sizes; all shapes and colours*. It is easy to read, colourful and informative with great appeal for men.[33]

Information that aims to communicate risks to patients, should cover the harmful effect(s) itself, the probability of it occurring, how to minimise this risk if possible, and what actions to take in the event of a problem arising. So:

- put the most important information first
- include information about benefits too
- use the right words that readers can understand
- use numbers appropriately to convey risk (*see* p. 74 for more about how to communicate risk effectively).

The Plain English Campaign and the Royal National Institute of the Blind (RNIB) are useful sources of advice and guidance on writing about health topics for various readerships.[34,35]

Online resources

Guiding individual or groups of patients on the use of appropriate websites will be of value. Health on Net gives details of its accreditation service for websites that adhere to its code of practice to help standardise the reliability of medical and health information available (www.hon.ch/HONcode). The StaRNeT website assessment tool (SWAT) is a rating instrument to evaluate general practice websites providing health information for patients.[36] When you can print off relevant pages from sites of proven quality you feel safe recommending the sites to patients (e.g. www.patient.co.uk, run by two GPs in Northumberland). Patients' awareness of NHS Direct Online services for instance, such as BestTreatments (www.besttreatments.co.uk) and the self help guide (www.nhsdirect.nhs.uk), are low and could be encouraged. You can signpost patients to online resources of self care support networks (e.g. that of the UK-based Addison's disease self help group www.adshg.org.uk contains practical information, and stories of patients' experiences). One of the websites with a listing of the largest number of self care support groups is www.ukselfhelp.info. Some websites are for both health professionals and the general public (e.g. Midwives Online www.midwivesonline.com). The MyPil resource at www.mypil.com provides patient information leaflets in several languages, such as Hindi, Urdu and Bengali.

New IT technology

The National Programme for Information Technology should fulfil people's wish to become involved in, and informed about, their care, through readily available information about health services, particular diseases and conditions and their own specific care plans.[37] Patients will have their own personal online health organiser, HealthSpace, that they can use to record personal health details such as blood pressure. It will incorporate a 'find' facility, allowing patients to look up reliable health related information, and provide guidance and information on healthy lifestyles. It will store self care programmes such as for stopping smoking or managing diabetes.

If patients with health concerns utilise the range of health information available, they may no longer need to become patients by consulting a health professional. They can investigate health issues themselves, before, or instead of, a consultation. A computer literate person may be able to find a satisfactory answer to their health issues online or on digital TV; many people will still need the expertise from health professionals they trust to interpret the data and information for them.[38]

Revising your personal development plan to focus on supporting self care for patients

Many health professionals and managers use personal learning plans as a way of thinking about planning and managing their learning: to consider their practice, define their learning needs and review progress. You probably have your own template already, but if not take a look at www.pdptoolkit.co.uk.

Tool 10 is a simple model for assessing your own educational needs in respect of supporting self care. Tool 17 helps you check that the learning you have identified is really a priority for you or your practice. Educational needs in this instance will encompass evolving a culture of self care in your practice or workplace, as well as the knowledge and skills for any particular role or responsibility you hold.

Use a range of methods to identify your training or information needs. No one method will give you reliable information about gaps in your knowledge, skills or attitudes. You can become more aware of your current gaps in knowledge, or your strengths and weaknesses in relation to supporting self care by:

- self-assessment and reflection
- peer review from work colleagues
- asking patients, users and non-users of your service
- comparing the way you support self care against best practice
- asking colleagues from different disciplines about shortfalls in how your work interfaces with theirs.

Demonstrating your competence in relation to self care through a personal portfolio

Maintain a portfolio that describes the evidence of what you have learnt, starting from your personal plan arising from your learning objectives, the process of gaining the knowledge or skills and the demonstration of your competence – with respect to supporting self care, in this instance. Such a portfolio may be useful in your annual appraisal or re-accreditation of your professional qualifications, to obtain credits for Prior Learning with higher degree courses at universities, or to prove experience and competence for a new role or cataloguing within the NHS Knowledge and Skills Framework component of Agenda for Change.

The steps in portfolio based learning are:[39]

- identifying significant experiences to serve as important sources of learning
- reflecting on the learning that arose from those experiences
- demonstrating that learning in practice
- analysing the portfolio (*see* Box 5.14) and identifying further learning needs and ways in which these needs can be met.

> **Box 5.14:** Your portfolio
>
> Your portfolio will have a varied content:
>
> - workload logs
> - case descriptions
> - videos
> - audiotapes
> - patient surveys
> - research surveys
> - audit projects
> - report of a change or innovation
> - notes from formal teaching sessions or action learning set
> - commentaries on published literature or books
> - records of critical incidents and learning points
> - patient narratives or stories.

Analysis of the experiences and learning opportunities should show demonstrable learning outcomes and any further educational plan to meet educational needs or development still outstanding. Much of the learning emanating from a portfolio is from individual reflection and self-critique in the analysis stage.

Being competent as a health professional in supporting self care

Developing competency: novice to expert

Competence is about being 'able to perform the tasks and roles required to the expected standard'.[40] So, knowledge and skill are components of competence. Capability is a term that describes 'what a person can think or do'. Whether or not a person's capability makes them competent in a particular job such as being a practice nurse depends on them being able to meet the requirements of that job.[41] Capability implies that individuals can develop sustainable abilities that allow them to adapt to a changing environment and react appropriately to unfamiliar situations.

You should set out the evidence of your competence in your portfolio to show that you know about self care, know how to promote and support it, can show how you are competent to promote and support it, and how you have done so (your performance).[42]

The standard expected to be able to judge someone as 'competent' will vary with their experience and level of responsibility, and take into account the need to keep up-to-date with changes in practice. Different people will have varied expectations of what counts as competence – managers, staff, individuals, patients, clients, etc.

There can be a gap between competence (what a person can do) and performance (what a person actually does). This gap can be caused by personal matters such as an individual's attitude or personality or mood, environmental factors such as workload, time pressures or working conditions, or situational factors such as a lack of resources or support.

You will become aware of what self care means, how to support self care, the risks and benefits, and how you can expect patients to practise it. As you become more familiar with the concept of self care and how various patients can apply it with their various health conditions and diverse circumstances, you will become competent at supporting self care. With more experience and continued learning and reflection about what works in supporting self care for patients, and what does not, you will become expert. This progress is described in Box 5.15.

Box 5.15: A health professional's competence in relation to supporting self care

Aware
Understands the importance of self care in generating health and wellbeing benefits to all people, and those with minor ailments and/or long term conditions. Able to signpost people who would benefit from self care to appropriate resources and an appropriate health professional.

$\downarrow$

Competent
In addition to the descriptor of being 'aware' of self care:

- has the knowledge and skills and positive attitude to promote and support self care for all patients consulting them in their everyday work role
- knows role within the practice team and is good team member in respect of self care, adhering to agreed messages and protocols
- is pro-active in supporting self care to all patients at every opportunity over and above the specific reason for their consultation
- takes into account self care activities the patient may be undertaking that might impact on a particular consultation (e.g. consuming OTC medicines, alternative therapies, healthy lifestyle behaviours)

$\downarrow$

Expert
In addition to the descriptor of being 'competent' in self care:

- has an intuitive grasp of the benefits of self care support and applies expert knowledge and skills about self care to patients at every opportunity
- knows how and has skills to initiate self care support activities and protocols with other members of the practice team and attached community nurses, AHPs and pharmacists
- knows how and has skills to initiate self care activities for the local population of the practice.

	Unconscious	Conscious
Competence	Unconscious competence	Conscious competence
Incompetence	Unconscious incompetence	Conscious incompetence

Figure 5.4: The stages of competence.

Conscious or unconscious competence should be your goal

You should strive to be consciously or unconsciously competent – the two upper quadrants in Figure 5.4. It is unprofessional to be consciously incompetent and a failure of your review of evidence for your portfolio to be unconsciously incompetent.

Matching your knowledge and skills to the Agenda for Change Framework

The NHS Knowledge and Skills Framework (KSF) covers everyone, except doctors working in general practice, who is employed by PCTs, and those working in general practice where practice employers take up the option under Agenda for Change.[43–46] The type and extent of knowledge and skills that define specific roles in supporting self care apply to most members of a general practice team. The six generic core dimensions of everyone's roles listed in Box 5.16 demonstrate how relevant they are to self care support.

Box 5.16: Brief descriptions of the six core dimensions of the NHS Knowledge and Skills Framework as relevant to the promotion and support of self care[43]

1 *Communication*: consistently practise good communication skills
2 *Personal and people development*: develop own skills and knowledge and provide information and advice to others to help their development
3 *Health, safety and security*: assist in maintaining others' health, safety and security
4 *Service development*: contribute to the improvement of NHS services
5 *Quality improvement*: demonstrate personal commitment to quality improvement, offering others advice and support
6 *Equality and diversity*: act in ways that support equality and value diversity

---

Illustrative example of evidence to demonstrate that you are competent at enabling patients to adopt self care

You might use or adapt the following example to gather evidence that you are performing well in relation to the promotion of self care by someone with back pain.[47]

Focus: complementary medicine, back pain, clinical care; evidence based practice

> **Case study 5.1**
> Ms Hope consults you (you might be a GP, practice nurse, pharmacist, physiotherapist or occupational therapist for this case study) to ask for advice about what complementary therapies she might try to help her back pain, as conventional medicines she has tried (paracetamol and ibuprofen) do not give her enough pain relief. She wants to know if acupuncture, glucosamine or massage are safe and worth trying.

Stage 1: Set your aspirations for good practice

The excellent health professional:

- knows about the nature and reliability of common treatments, whether they are conventional or complementary treatments
- maintains their knowledge and skills, and is aware of their limits of competence.

Stage 2: Set the standards for your outcomes

Outcomes might include:

- a protocol in relation to self care of back pain
- a strategy that is implemented in respect of self care support (for back pain)
- meeting recommended standards in respect of self care support.

Be able to explain the evidence base for interventions (conventional NHS care and self care) that give benefits for low back pain.

Stage 3A: Identify your learning needs

- Self-assess your knowledge of the benefits/risks of complementary treatments, especially acupuncture, glucosamine and massage for back pain.
- Try to find reliable evidence about the complementary interventions in question within 5 minutes – either from the PC in your consulting room or a nearby book. Do you know the websites or publication to access easily for the evidence base?
- Once you have learnt enough about the effectiveness of these interventions (*see* Stage 4) explain the evidence to the patient – and then ask for feedback from the patient as to whether they understood your explanation or have any more questions.

Stage 3B: Identify your service needs

> Any of the needs assessment exercises in 3A may also reveal service needs.

- Check if there is any patient literature about self care of back pain in the waiting room or consulting rooms. Does it cover complementary treatments? Do you or others in the team know any websites covering self care, to which patients can be directed ?
- Find out what local services exist to provide acupuncture or massage through the NHS or privately.

Stage 4: Make and carry out a learning and action plan
- Read up about the effectiveness of interventions for acute and chronic back pain from a reliable source.
- Discuss with two patients, patient literature that you have accessed from reliable websites as to the relevance and readability of the material.

Stage 5: Document your learning, competence, performance and standards of service delivery
- Place photocopies of the evidence for treatments for back pain in your portfolio so that you can refer to it in future if other patients ask you the same questions about the effectiveness of complementary treatments.
- Include copies of relevant patient literature.

> **Case study 5.1 continued**
> Ms Hope listened to the evidence you relayed that the effectiveness of acupuncture and massage is unknown as regards back pain, and that there is some evidence that glucosamine may be beneficial for osteoarthritis. She decided to give acupuncture a go, as it seemed reasonably safe to do so, and found that her pain subsided considerably as a result of her self organised care.

Communicating risk to patients in relation to self care

In order for people to make well-informed decisions about their self care or medical management, they need to understand the risks and benefits resulting from choices that they make.[48] They need to compare those risks with other risks in their lives.

Your advice to a patient must fit with the way they look at the world, and take into account their personality and understanding. The language you use to describe risk is as important as the way you rate and present it. Risk is the probability that a hazard will give rise to harm. But the extent to which a person judges that the harmful outcome is likely to occur and the extent to which they judge the likely outcome to be harmful are subjective. Personality type will influence the way in which risk is allowed to influence behaviour. Some people have a tendency to optimism despite the evidence. Pessimistic people tend to assume that risks are greater than they really are, maybe as a self protection mechanism.

Misperceptions about risk

On the whole, people tend to be over-optimistic about the risks they face. Most smokers acknowledge the connection between smoking and disease but generally underestimate the extent to which they feel that risk applies to them. If asked to estimate the risk we feel we face from heart disease, for example, or being involved in a car accident there will be a bias towards optimism. Outcomes with a high probability tend to be underestimated, whereas the risk from rare events such as nuclear accidents tends to be overestimated.

So a misperception exists. People tend towards the illusion of relative invulnerability, even complacency where more common risks exist, and towards unnecessary concern for less likely, but more newsworthy, events. Since perception of risk is a prerequisite for changes in behaviour, misplaced optimism may hinder preventative action. An increased sense of risk, especially when combined with low expectations for being able to deal with that risk, may provoke a 'helplessness reaction' and obstruct intentions to adapt or modify behaviour. This has implications for the way doctors and nurses talk to patients about risk in an attempt to modify unhealthy behaviour and promote self care.

Tolerating risk

We tend to build in an element of uncertainty to our life to prevent boredom or to increase reward. Our risk 'thermostat' is not set at zero. The setting of the 'thermostat' varies from one individual to another and for one individual over time, as their circumstances and life events change. We also consider the effect that that harm would have on us if it were to occur. Variously known as the 'dread factor' or 'fright factor', these can be more important than the statistical probability of occurrence.

Communicating risk to patients

Patients may modify their own behaviour as their perception of risks and benefits changes, rather than in response to your exhortations as a health professional. A person who feels that change will have no effect on the inevitability of a poor outcome may be as unlikely to change as one unrealistically optimistic about his or her chances. What influences the reaction of any individual to information about risk are that:

- the impact of the anticipated outcome must matter to them
- the action required to influence such an outcome must fit their view of the 'world'
- they must agree that a particular outcome is possible
- the source of the information must be trustworthy.

You need to find a way to communicate risks as well as benefits from OTC medicines – as in Box 5.17. You might use a visual scale to demonstrate risk to patients. For instance, an online risk calculator can help GPs and specialist diabetes nurses assess cardiovascular risk in patients with type 2 diabetes. You could look at this together with the patient.[49]

Box 5.17: Example of risks from complementary medicines

There can be potentially dangerous consequences from combining OTC medicines with prescribed drugs. For example, the herbal drug St John's wort reacts adversely with some commonly prescribed drugs such as warfarin, oral contraceptives and some antidepressant drugs.

Explaining the level of risk

There is an inbuilt difficulty in using probability to measure risk for anyone who is not good with numbers. Is a side-effect of a drug with a risk of 1:10 000 something we need to be concerned about? What if there is a risk of death of 50% from that side-effect, or a 12% risk of impotence?

The way in which a consequence is presented is termed its 'frame', and this can affect the choices patients make, clouding or enhancing the true consequences of an action.

Would you choose an intervention with a 40% failure rate or a 60% success rate? The actual risk of the two interventions is the same – but many would choose the one 'framed' in terms of gains. Health professionals use framing almost instinctively to discourage patients from certain activities, framing in terms of negative outcomes while still giving correct facts.

Time management

Time pressures are a barrier to health professionals encouraging patients to take more part in decision making and supporting self care.[26,48,50]

The many ways to manage your time better fall into three main categories:

1 *reducing the amount of work to be done* by refusing it in the first place, delegating it, or doing less of it. Reviewing how work is delegated from GPs to nurses, and from practice nurses to health care assistants perhaps?
2 *doing work more quickly* by doing it less thoroughly or processing it more efficiently. Making more use of the computer and working more efficiently perhaps?
3 *allowing more time for a particular piece of work* with less time pressure on completing it – altering the way you book patients perhaps?

Prioritise your time: do not allow yourself or others to waste it

Be clear about your goals in your work. Then structure sufficient time around those priorities. When an activity arises over which you have choice, match it against your goals. If it takes you further away from your goals, then refuse to take it on, but if it coincides with your goals, consider whether you have time to fit it in.

Make sure that you spend your quality time doing the most important or complex jobs. A high-priority task has to be done, a medium-priority job may be delegated, and a low-priority task should only be done if you have no medium- or high-priority tasks waiting. The majority of your time should be devoted to pursuing your most important goals, and a small proportion of your time spent on less important matters.

Try to allow at least 10% of your time for dealing with unexpected tasks. In the unlikely event that everything goes smoothly and you do not need the extra time, it will be a bonus to have that additional space to catch up on your backlog, or simply spend that time talking to people about how they are feeling or what they are doing.

Delegate whatever and however you can

Only accept delegated work if you have the necessary skills, time and experience. If you are in a position to delegate work and responsibilities, decide what only *you* can do, and delegate as much as possible of the rest to others. If you are more usually on the receiving end of delegated work, try to make sure you understand what is required, and that you have the time, skills and experience, before agreeing or acquiescing to taking on the new work.

Self care for you too as a health professional or manager

You cannot work effectively if you are over-pressured or under mental or emotional strain. Apply the principles and practice of self care to yourself too.

The problem with stress

Stress is equivalent to a person's perception of the pressure upon them, or the 'three-way relationship between demands on a person, that person's feelings about those demands, and their ability to cope with those demands'.[51] In other words, a particular event or task can be stressful for you one day but not on another – depending on how you are feeling and what other pressures are being exerted on you.

In general, stress occurs in situations where the workload is high, control over the workload is limited, and too little support or help is available. A moderate amount of stress is necessary to perform well at work and to maintain a zest for life; zero stress may lead to boredom, whereas too much stress over too long a period will render you indecisive, exhausted or 'burnt out'.

There are three types of responses to stress – physiological, psychological and behavioural reactions. The ways we respond depend on personal factors such as age, gender, personality, previous family and personal experiences, as well as coping ability and other organisational options.

Dealing with stress

The kind of practical methods people can use to cope with stress at work are:

- seeking support from colleagues
- sharing problems with colleagues
- adopting better time management practices
- more appropriate booking times for appointments and meetings
- increased protected time off-duty, limiting working hours to those for which contracted
- admitting doubts and worries to others
- achieving a better balance between work and home commitments.

Stress itself is not the damaging factor but rather your inability to cope with it. In a changing world, people need to learn new ways of coping. That way lies survival.

Seek support

People with the best social support interact well with other people, are able to cope with stress and are the least affected by it. Look at Tool 18 to consider the range of sources of support in your life. Be prepared to ask for help. That is not a sign of weakness or ignorance.

Balance your work and leisure time successfully

Timetable enough free time during your day to have space for rest and relaxation to counteract stresses and strains. Try and complete work activities within your normal working hours, so that you have enough time for non-work-related activities in your life. Make regular time and space for yourself for fun, relaxation, hobbies and enjoying simple pleasures throughout your life as a *stress proofing* measure.

References

1. WONCA. *The European Definition Of General Practice/Family Medicine*. Barcelona: WONCA Europe; 2002.
2. Royal College of General Practitioners. *The Nature of General Medical Practice. Report from general practice 27*. London: Royal College of General Practitioners; 1996.
3. Grueninger U. *WONCA Tree*. Geneva: Swiss College of Family Medicine; 2004.
4. Critchlow M. *Enabling Self Care. Report on focus groups of patients with long term conditions, and healthcare professionals*. London: Health First; 2005.
5. Hargie ODW. *The Handbook of Communication Skills* (2e). London: Routledge; 1997.
6. Healthcare Commission. *Primary Care Trust: survey of patients 2005*. London: Healthcare Commission; 2005.
7. Kennedy A, Gask L, Rogers A. Training professionals to engage with and promote self-management. *Health Education Research*. 2005; **20**: 567–8.

8 Richards A, Barkham M, Cahill J et al. PHASE: a randomised, controlled trial of supervised self-help cognitive behavioural therapy in primary care. *British Journal of General Practice.* 2003; **53:** 764–70.

9 The Working in Partnership Programme. www.wipp.nhs.uk

10 Longo MF, Cohen DR, Hood K et al. Involving patients in primary care consultations: assessing preferences using discrete choice experiments. *British Journal of General Practice.* 2006; **56:** 35–42.

11 Jordan J, Ellis S and Chambers R. Defining shared decision making and concordance: are they one and the same? *Postgraduate Medical Journal.* 2002; **78:** 383–4.

12 Royal Pharmaceutical Society of Great Britain. *From Compliance to Concordance: achieving shared goals in medicine taking.* London: Royal Pharmaceutical Society of Great Britain; 1997.

13 Weiss M and Britten N. What is concordance? *Pharmaceutical Journal.* 2003; **271:** 493.

14 Medicines Partnership. www.medicines-partnership.org

15 Say R and Thomson R. The importance of patient preferences in treatment decisions – challenges for doctors. *British Medical Journal.* 2003; **327:** 542–5.

16 Myers G. *Doctor Prescribes, Patient Complies? A concordance skills workshop.* Medicines Partnership. London: Lambeth PCT; 2005.

17 www.medicines-partnership.org/professional-development/training-resources/catchphrases

18 Tim Scott. *Enterprising Use of IT – patient care IT system.* Derbyshire: The Imaginative Health Cluster; 2005. www.GPonline.com/full_enterprise_awards.cfm?ID=12343

19 Miller WR and Rollnick S. *Motivational Interviewing: preparing people for change* (2e). New York: The Guildford Press; 2002.

20 Bandura A. Health promotion by social cognitive means. *Health Education Behaviour.* 2004; **31:** 143–64.

21 Heron J. *Helping the Client.* London: Sage Publications; 2001.

22 Chambers R. Weighing up the best test of fitness. *The Sentinel.* 2005; **27 December:** 24.

23 Prochaska J, DiClemente C and Norcross J. In search of how people change. *American Psychologist.* 1992; **47:** 1102–14.

24 Eekhof JA, Knuistingh Neven A and Verheij TJM (eds). *Minor Ailments in Primary Care – an evidence-based approach.* London: Elsevier; 2005.

25 National Statistics. *Contraception and Sexual Health 2004/05.* National Statistics series OS no 28. www.statistics.gov.uk/statbase/Product.asp?vlnk=6988

26 Blenkinsopp A and Archer J. *Winter Ailments. A tutor manual.* Manchester: Centre for Pharmacy Postgraduate Education; 2000.

27 Bednall R, McRobbie D, Duncan J and Williams D. Identification of patients attending Accident and Emergency who may be suitable for treatment by a pharmacist. *Family Practice.* 2003; **20:** 54–7.

28 Blenkinsopp A and Bond C. *Over-the-counter Medication.* London: Board of Science, British Medical Association; 2005.

29 Committee on Safety of Medicines Working Group on Patient Information. *Always Read the Leaflet. Getting the best information with every medicine.* London: The Stationery Office; 2005.

30 Duman M. *Producing Patient Information. How to research, develop and produce effective information resources*. London: King's Fund; 2003.

31 Coulter A, Entwistle V and Gilbert D. *Informing Patients*. London: King's Fund; 1998.

32 Charnock D. *The DISCERN Handbook*. Oxford: Radcliffe Medical Press; 1998.

33 Banks I. *HGV Man – reducing all large sizes; all shapes and colours. Haynes Owners Workshop Manual*. Somerset: Haynes Publishing; 2005.

34 Plain English Campaign www.plainenglish.co.uk

35 Royal National Institute of the Blind. www.rnib.org.uk

36 Howitt A, Clement S, de Lusignan S et al. An evaluation of general practice websites in the UK. *Family Practice*. 2002; **19**: 547–56.

37 NHS Connecting for Health. *A Guide to the National Programme for Information Technology*. London: NHS Connecting for Health; 2005. www.connectingforhealth.nhs.uk

38 Sullivan F and Wyatt J. Is a consultation needed? ABC of health informatics. *British Medical Journal*. 2005; **331**: 625–7.

39 Royal College of General Practitioners. *Portfolio-based Learning in General Practice*. Occasional Paper 63. London: Royal College of General Practitioners; 1993.

40 Eraut M and du Boulay B. *Developing the Attributes of Medical Professional Judgement and Competence*. Sussex: University of Sussex; 2000. www.informatics.sussex.ac.uk/users/bend/doh

41 Fraser SW and Greenhalgh T. Coping with complexity: educating for capability. *British Medical Journal*. 2001; **323**: 799–802.

42 Davies H. Work based assessment. *BMJ Careers*. 2005; **20 August:** 88–9.

43 Department of Health. *The NHS Knowledge and Skills Framework*. London: Department of Health; 2004. www.dh.gov.uk

44 Department of Health. *Agenda for Change – what will it mean for you?* London: Department of Health; 2004. www.dh.gov.uk

45 Tavabie A and Chambers R. Making a case for the NHS Knowledge and Skills Framework to be applied in general practice: why exclude GPs and their practice teams? *Education for Primary Care*. 2004; **15**: 304–10.

46 Johnston J. 10 tips on moving to Agenda for Change. *Medeconomics*. 2005; **November:** 32–3.

47 Chambers R, Mohanna K, Wakley G and Wall D. *Demonstrating your Competence 1: healthcare teaching*. Oxford: Radcliffe Medical Press; 2004.

48 Mohanna K and Chambers R. *Risk Matters in Healthcare: communicating, explaining and managing risk*. Oxford: Radcliffe Medical Press; 2000.

49 Diabetes Trials Unit. www.dtu.ox.ac.uk

50 Edwards A, Elwyn G, Wood F et al. Shared decision making and risk communication in practice. *British Journal of General Practice*. 2005; **55**: 6–13.

51 Richards C. *The Health of Doctors*. London: King's Fund; 1989.

6

Getting organised for promoting and supporting self care as a pharmacy team

Alison Blenkinsopp

This chapter describes how you can get organised in a community pharmacy to design a strategy and implementation plan in relation to supporting self care. The outcome should be a culture whereby supporting self care is integral to all your developments and services making the most of local initiatives and the pharmacy contract. Pharmacists and the staff will promote and support self care as part of their everyday work in effective ways.

The community pharmacy is a natural hub for promoting and supporting self care. Integration of community pharmacy into primary care is closer to becoming a reality as a result of the new contractual frameworks for pharmacy and general practice. Pharmacy teams cannot promote self care in isolation from other health care professionals and their teams, and it is more important than ever that patients and the public receive consistent messages about self care. Look back at Chapters 3 and 4 to realise how the community pharmacist can be included in the PCT's and general medical practice's efforts at supporting self care. Community pharmacy teams can follow the algorithm in Figure 4.1 in a similar way to that of general medical practice teams, to build a self care culture and focus on worthwhile self care support interventions.

Requirements and opportunities: the community pharmacy contract

The community pharmacy contract promotes the involvement of community pharmacy teams in self care.[1] The contractual framework has three types of service:

- *essential*: provided by all pharmacies, with national specification and funding
- *advanced*: provided by accredited pharmacies, with national specification and funding
- *enhanced* (with national template and locally commissioned).

There are three interconnected *essential* services that directly concern self care and will be provided by all pharmacies (*see* Table 6.1).

Supporting self care

The 'Supporting self care' essential service covers both self-limiting problems and long term conditions.

Table 6.1: Essential services and self care

Essential service	Description	Focus	What's new?
Support for self care	Provision of advice and support by pharmacy staff to enable people to derive maximum benefit from caring for themselves and their families	Support for self management of self-limiting and long term conditions	Recording of pharmacist's contribution to care
Signposting	Provision of information to people who require further support, advice or treatment which cannot be provided by the pharmacy. Where appropriate, this may take the form of a referral	Other health and social care providers, and support organisations	Opportunities for referral to health and social resources more formal than before
Promotion of healthy lifestyles (public health)	Provision of opportunistic advice on lifestyle and public health issues to patients receiving prescriptions and proactive participation in national/local campaigns to promote public health messages	General pharmacy visitors and 'hard to reach' groups. People presenting prescriptions for diabetes, those at risk of CHD, particularly those with hypertension, those who smoke and those who are overweight	Brief interventions in long term conditions; targeted using prescriptions; participation in health campaigns now compulsory

Self-limiting problems

Commonly referred to by health professionals as 'minor ailments', self-limiting problems will resolve with or without treatment. The essential service 'Support for self care' incorporates the traditional community pharmacy work of responding to requests for advice about symptoms, recommending OTC treatments and advice on home remedies, and referring to another health professional where needed. The new element is the requirement for record keeping for certain transactions: 'For patients known to the pharmacy staff, records of advice given, products purchased or referrals made *will* [our emphasis] be made on a patient's pharmacy record when the pharmacist deems it to be of clinical significance'.[1]

This requirement for record keeping is the first time that there has been an explicit acknowledgement of the role of pharmacy advice and treatment for self-limiting conditions within the NHS. It is also the first time that community pharmacy's contribution to clinical care has been documented. Its long term value will be in the implementation and whether pharmacists and other members of the primary care team use the documentation in follow-up. These records will become increasingly important as more treatments for intermittent and long term conditions switch from prescription only to OTC status. Auditing records for what advice has been given, and how, will enable pharmacists to review their standards of care and safety and make plans for improvement.

People seek advice in pharmacies about a wide range of health problems. Pharmacy staff have always performed a triaging role in advising when self management is appropriate and when further expert advice is needed. Community pharmacies are one source of advice and treatment about minor illness in primary care. Patients might see their GP, a nurse in a general practice-based nurse-led 'minor illness clinic' or NHS Walk-in-Centre (WIC) or seek advice from the NHS Direct range of services. The number of different settings and health professionals involved increases the risk of people receiving differing advice. The PART model (prevention, await resolution, relief of symptoms, toleration of symptoms) is used in Table 6.2 to explore the factors influencing these differences.[2]

In some areas, ways of increasing consistency between health professionals are being found, such as shared information leaflets for patients (*see* example in Box 6.1).

Table 6.2: Potential for different messages about self care

Advice area	Content	Influencing factors
Prevention	Advice on action/s to take to prevent recurrence	Access to current evidence
Await resolution	Evidence of natural history and timescale of condition	Patient experience and preferences
	Evidence of effectiveness of treatment or other advice	Access to current evidence
		Level of consensus between professionals
Relief of symptoms	Evidence of effectiveness of treatment or other advice	Patient experience and preferences
		Access to current evidence
		Level of consensus between professionals
Toleration of symptoms	Natural course of symptom/condition	Access to current evidence
	Expected time to improvement or resolution	Level of consensus between professionals
Triggers for referral	Specific symptoms and/or duration of problem	Professional decisions about what requires an 'urgent' appointment

> **Box 6.1:** Shared patient leaflets on minor ailments for pharmacies and practices
>
> Walsall PCT links the health promotion topics agreed by the PCT for the essential services public health component of the pharmacy contract, with information provided in GP surgeries. Having decided that minor ailments would be a good topic for the winter months the PCT used patient leaflets on cough, earache and sore throat produced as part of their 'IMPACT' programme. A poster was also produced for use within pharmacies and practices. The leaflets explain the cause of the problem, why antibiotics are not needed, self care actions that can be taken, and tips on when to see the doctor.

Community pharmacy minor ailment scheme

In many areas, pharmacy advice and treatment for self-limiting problems has been incorporated into locally-commissioned NHS services, as community pharmacy minor ailment schemes (MAS). This increases patients' access to services and improves the management of workload in general practice by transferring some work to other professionals. The MAS service can be commissioned by PCTs as an *enhanced* service in the pharmacy contract. Patients who are exempt from NHS prescription charges receive any treatment needed from a locally agreed formulary, free of charge. Examples of ailments included in existing schemes are given in Box 6.2.

> **Box 6.2:** Conditions included in NHS minor ailments schemes
> - Backache, sprains and strains
> - Colds
> - Conjunctivitis
> - Constipation
> - Cough
> - Diarrhoea
> - Earache
> - Haemorrhoids
> - Hay fever
> - Head lice
> - Headache and fever
> - Heartburn and indigestion
> - Insect bites and stings
> - Mild eczema and dermatitis
> - Minor fungal infections of the skin
> - Mouth ulcers
> - Nappy rash
> - Sore throat

- Teething
- Threadworms
- Thrush

Source: Pharmaceutical Services Negotiating Committee Enhanced service template: minor ailment schemes[3]

Conditions included in a scheme are agreed between local GPs, community pharmacists and the PCT. Eligibility for patients to participate is also decided locally. Schemes can be open only to patients who are referred during a request for a GP appointment, or through self-referral. The pharmacy contractor receives a locally negotiated consultation fee plus, where a medicine is supplied, the cost of the medicine.

Some schemes include ailments where the only effective treatment is a POM and use a patient group direction (PGD) to enable the pharmacist to supply it. The legal definition of a PGD is 'a written instruction for the sale, supply and/or administration of named medicines in an identified clinical situation. It applies to groups of patients who may not be individually identified before presenting for treatment'.[4] PGDs are appropriate to manage a specific treatment episode where the supply and administration of a medicine is necessary, as in first contact services and urgent or emergency care. The commonest examples are topical antibacterials to treat conjunctivitis (although chloramphenicol eye drops have since been switched from prescription to OTC availability) and oral antibacterials to treat uncomplicated urinary tract infection (at the time of writing the outcome of a consultation for the switch of trimethoprim to OTC availability was awaited) and for impetigo. In some areas the MAS is used specifically to divert people who are known to need a treatment that is a POM (*see* example in Box 6.3).

Box 6.3: Taunton Deane MAS

Taunton Deane PCT focused its community pharmacy minor ailment scheme on conditions that could otherwise only be treated by a GP. Following introduction of the new General Medical Services (nGMS) contract, fewer practices were open on Saturday mornings and with the shift to out of hours (OOH) providers there was concern that attendances at accident and emergency services (A&E) might rise for common conditions.[5] All of the 18 local pharmacies participated. The PCT had considered which were the commonest conditions in calls to NHS Direct (conjunctivitis and urinary tract infections were in the top ten) and consulted locally about which conditions to include. The list included conjunctivitis, vaginal thrush, urinary tract infection, impetigo and hay fever.

In the first year there were 560 consultations, with Saturday showing the highest demand. Just over half of the medicines supplied on PGD were for conjunctivitis, 20% for urinary tract infection and 9% for impetigo. Sixteen of the 18 local pharmacies were involved in consultations (ranging from fewer

> than ten to over 80 per pharmacy). The PCT has continued discussions with the OOH providers and A&E about commonly presenting conditions that could be managed in pharmacies.

A particular advantage of pharmacy MAS is that they can provide NHS cover when local GP surgeries are closed at weekends and patients might otherwise go to A&E.

Providing ready access to emergency hormonal contraception (EHC) is now an important role of community pharmacies; this has reduced attendances at A&E.[6] A systematic review concluded that access to EHC had improved and that women rated the pharmacy supply positively.[7] Although EHC is available for purchase OTC the cost precludes its use for many women. Some PCTs have established a scheme to improve access to emergency contraception, where the supply is made from community pharmacies without charge to the patient using a PGD.

Community pharmacists also contribute to OOH services, particularly by providing telephone advice for patients who have been triaged (see Box 6.4).

> **Box 6.4:** Out of hours advice from a multidisciplinary team in primary care
>
> Telephone advice from a multidisciplinary team comprising doctors, nurses and community pharmacists is provided from Fylde Coast Medical Services (FCMS), an urban OOH centre in Blackpool. Over 20 of the area's 160 pharmacists participate in the service.
>
> FCMS has some 50 000 patient contacts per year. In addition to OOH medical services, the centre includes emergency social services, night nursing, emergency dentistry, mental health crisis team and palliative care equipment. The centre also provides OOH medical support for the local NHS WIC.
>
> An audit of patient consultations showed that 45% were for minor ailments, the commonest of these being: cough (32%), temperature (19%), sore throat (19%), earache (12%), diarrhoea (8%) and head lice (5%). Analysis of the prescriptions written for minor ailments at FCMS prior to the introduction of the multidisciplinary service in 2003 showed that 46% were for non-prescription medicines. Work has identified which patients can be streamed to the pharmacist or nurse rather than the GP. In addition to providing telephone advice, pharmacists can supply medicines for minor ailments to patients who visit the centre.

Pharmacists' role in supporting self care in long term conditions

Community pharmacists can 'do more to help patients, keep them out of hospital and educate them and their carers about medication'.[8] The Department of Health public health strategy for the 'health promoting pharmacy' aims to 'improve the health of people with long term conditions by helping them with their medicines, promoting healthy lifestyles, supporting self care, signposting to other services and working closely with community matrons and case managers'.[9]

The contribution that community pharmacists could make is summarised in Figure 6.1.

The pyramid represents people with long term conditions, where 70–80% can take care of their condition with a small amount of support from professionals. Pharmacist input at Level 1 includes health promotion and opportunistic counselling, practical help with medicines use, and advising on the appropriate use of OTC medicines. These activities are covered by the *essential* services of support for self care and public health.

In the middle of the pyramid at Level 2 are the people whose long term condition needs more support from health professionals. Their asthma or diabetes might be more difficult to control for example.

At the top of the pyramid at Level 3 are the people who need the most intense level of support from the health service. These patients may have co-morbidities and conditions such as heart failure, chronic obstructive pulmonary disease and diabetes with complications. These patients have exacerbations of their condition that lead to multiple admissions to hospital.

Working at Levels 2 and 3 in the pyramid in Figure 6.1 relates to *advanced* and *enhanced* community pharmacy services. The example in Box 6.5 shows the service model that has been used in diabetes.

Box 6.5: Integrated support for people with diabetes

Hillingdon PCT, working with a private sector company, Pharmacy Alliance, designed a community pharmacy based programme for people with type 1 and type 2 diabetes, who were receiving antidiabetic medication. The community pharmacists provide a medicines support service to these patients, and facilitate optimal disease management and monitoring, in collaboration with GPs and other health care professionals. Pharmacists invite patients to take part and gain their consent to participate in the programme. The patient's random blood glucose, haemoglobin A_{1c} (HbA_{1c}), total cholesterol, blood pressure, body mass index (BMI) and waist measurement are taken and recorded. The patient then completes two questionnaires that assess their information needs and explore their beliefs about medicines. The pharmacist provides advice in response to the patient's answers. Where the pharmacist identifies a need that cannot be met by the pharmacy, the patient is referred to their GP. The patient returns for a review at two-monthly intervals. Patients receiving the service have shown improvements in all clinical measures and in their understanding of their condition and medication.

Asthma is another area where community pharmacy can potentially make a large contribution. Research conducted by Asthma UK found that 'people with asthma would appreciate more support and advice from their local pharmacist: for example, parents have told us that they see pharmacists as a valuable source of information about their child's asthma'.[10] Two examples of community pharmacy-based support for asthma are described in Box 6.6.

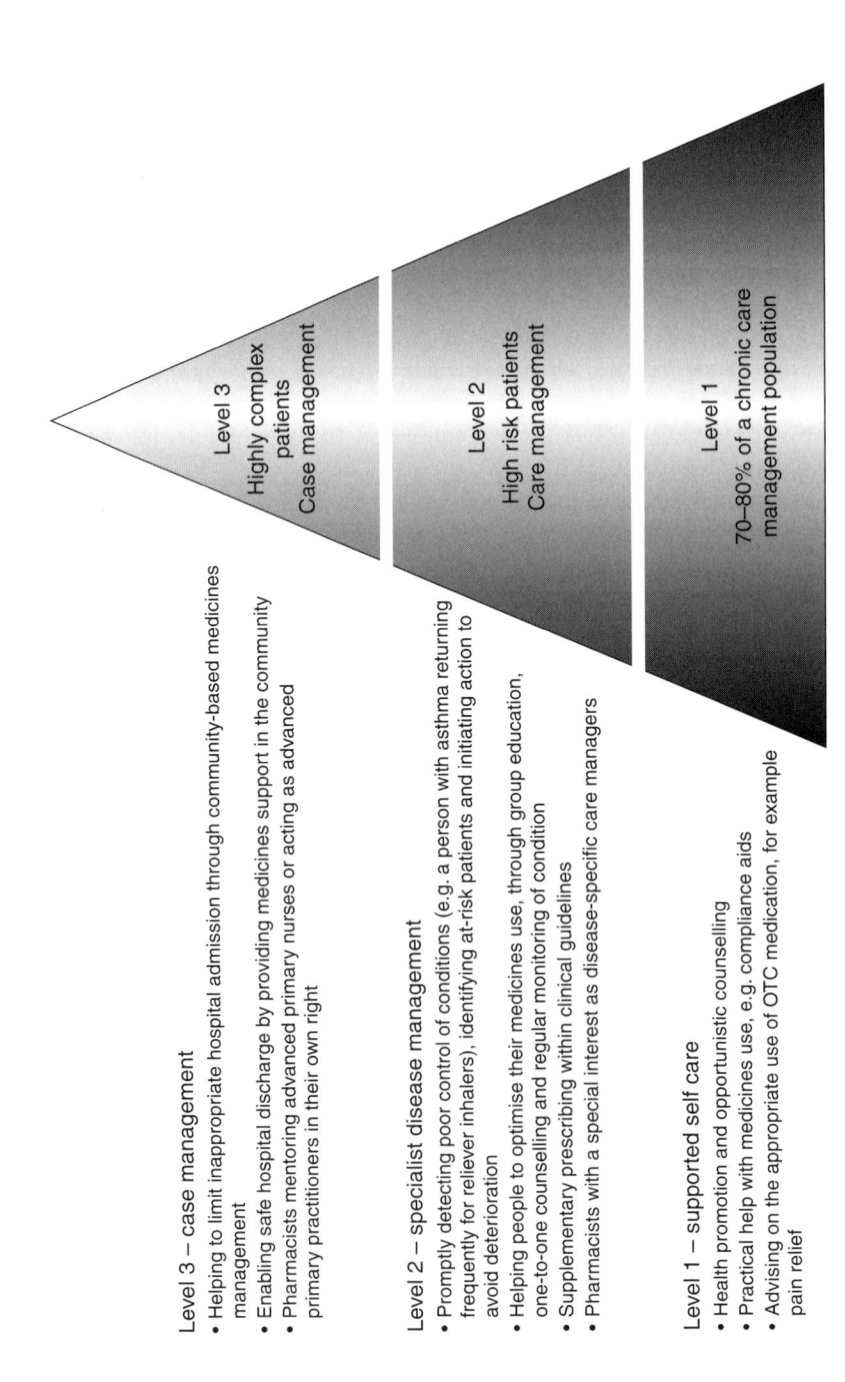

Level 3 – case management
- Helping to limit inappropriate hospital admission through community-based medicines management
- Enabling safe hospital discharge by providing medicines support in the community
- Pharmacists mentoring advanced primary nurses or acting as advanced primary practitioners in their own right

Level 2 – specialist disease management
- Promptly detecting poor control of conditions (e.g. a person with asthma returning frequently for reliever inhalers), identifying at-risk patients and initiating action to avoid deterioration
- Helping people to optimise their medicines use, through group education, one-to-one counselling and regular monitoring of condition
- Supplementary prescribing within clinical guidelines
- Pharmacists with a special interest as disease-specific care managers

Level 1 – supported self care
- Health promotion and opportunistic counselling
- Practical help with medicines use, e.g. compliance aids
- Advising on the appropriate use of OTC medication, for example pain relief

Figure 6.1: Community pharmacy's contribution in the care of people with long term conditions. Adapted from Department of Health.[11,12]

> **Box 6.6:** Asthma consultations in community pharmacies
>
> Boots, in collaboration with Asthma UK, have introduced an asthma service, initially in 50 of its stores across England. All pharmacy staff including health care assistants and dispensers have been trained to identify whether people's symptoms are well controlled, by asking three questions recommended by the Royal College of Physicians that focus on nocturnal and daytime symptoms, and whether these disturb sleep or curb daily activities. People are offered a ten-minute appointment with a specially trained pharmacist, and receive advice on managing their treatment and symptoms more effectively. Consultations cover inhaler technique, medicines management and lifestyle advice such as coping with coughs, colds or hay fever.
>
> Improving treatment compliance among patients with asthma was the aim of a pilot by the Moss Pharmacy company. The service was offered initially by eight of the company's pharmacies and involved pharmacists developing an asthma action plan for a patient, reviewing and educating the patient's inhaler technique, and monitoring the patient for six months. The pharmacist tackled compliance problems, or difficulties with inhaler technique, and any issues that could not be resolved were referred to GPs. Patients found to have uncontrolled symptoms, drug interactions or needing dose adjustment were also referred to the GP. Actions taken by the pharmacist were recorded in the patient's care plan.

One mechanism for community pharmacists to provide input to long term conditions is the *advanced* service of medicines use review (MUR).[1] The consultation for MUR can be used to ask trigger questions which may identify the need for further support, as in the asthma example above.

Pharmacies can contribute to long term condition management by providing accessible monitoring tests. The example relayed in Box 6.7 shows how this can work. A major challenge is the integration of pharmacy test results with GP records so that work is not duplicated, and information can be accessed by others who need it.

> **Box 6.7:** Greater Manchester High Street testing pilot
>
> Twenty-two pharmacies in Stockport, Oldham, Salford and Ashton, Leigh and Wigan PCTs, in a pilot public/private sector collaboration regularly monitor patients with diabetes and/or coronary heart disease. The pilot is sponsored by the Department of Health and supported by Pharmacy Alliance. Participating pharmacies include independents, regional multiples and national multiples. The pharmacists complete a specific training programme and the premises' facilities are upgraded with NHS support. Patients can choose whether to continue using existing services or the new services. Those that choose the pharmacy option are invited by their pharmacist for an initial consultation. A

patient history is taken and tests are performed by the pharmacist prior to a consultation with the patient. Measures regularly taken include:

- total cholesterol/high density lipoprotein (HDL)/triglycerides and low density lipoprotein (LDL)
- HbA_{1c}
- blood pressure
- weight (height), BMI and waist measurement.

The consultation covers the impact that medication, lifestyle, diet and activity can have on the patient's condition, and uses the test results to illustrate what changes can be made. Patients are seen at least twice a year. Exceptionally, the pharmacist may need to refer the patient back to their GP for urgent review. The pilot aims to promote greater collaboration between community pharmacists, GPs and other local healthcare providers. Data gathered in the consultation are relayed online to be inserted into the patient record and the GP's QOF record.[6]

Equipment selection, staff training, quality control, external quality assurance and performance management all form part of a governance system.

Promotion of healthy lifestyles (public health)

The *essential* service includes the pharmacy participating in locally endorsed campaigns each year together with prescription-linked interventions.

Local healthy lifestyles campaigns

Pharmacies are required by the contract to participate in up to six campaigns each year, using materials provided by the PCT.[1] Topics are agreed locally and the PCT is responsible for obtaining leaflets and other materials for the campaign. So, consistent information is provided from pharmacies and other locations participating in the campaigns. Nominating a lead per pharmacy and the promotion of healthy lifestyles is a business opportunity (*see* Box 6.8).

Box 6.8: Essential service – promoting healthy lifestyles and public health

Having one person to co-ordinate the receipt and display of leaflets and posters, and brief other staff on each topic could reduce the workload on the pharmacist as well as build public health skills in staff.

Linking pharmacy window displays with the current campaign topic promotes the pharmacy as a centre for health advice and draws people into the pharmacy, increasing requests for advice and information.

Prescription-linked interventions

Pharmacists are asked to target patients with diabetes, CHD and hypertension for brief interventions relating to their lifestyle, according to the patient's needs. Flexibility is envisaged in the advice offered, but might focus on smoking cessation, physical activity and diet. Record keeping will 'be in a form that facilitates audit of the provision of the service and follow-up with the patient who has been given advice'.[1]

Making links with the *signposting* service and prescription-linked interventions is important, for example, so that patients can be made aware of relevant local services. Pharmacists and their staff need to know about local availability. For example, a wide range of physical activity options exists, and the level of activity can be matched to the patient's capacity. Many of these are subsidised or provided free of charge by local councils or through local strategic partnerships. Some examples are given in Box 6.9.

Box 6.9: Examples of local physical activity resources
- *Guided walks*: graded walks of different intensity that can be matched to individual ability and used by adults and families
- *'Green gyms'*: local projects e.g. clearing ground in conservation areas
- *Chair-based exercise*: suitable where balance and mobility are limited
- *Tai Chi*: gentle exercise that improves balance and may help to prevent falls
- *Swimming*: specific sessions sometimes offered, e.g. for pregnant women and for people with arthritis

---

Local partnerships are leading multi-agency health improvement schemes. The 'Up for it?' programme described in Box 6.10 is an example of a community-wide scheme in which community pharmacy plays a part, integrated with other key local players.

Box 6.10: 'Up for it?' programme

The 'Up for it' programme is a health and lifestyle membership scheme that aims to motivate behavioural and lifestyle change. It was set up by the Blantyre/North Hamilton Social Inclusion Partnership (SIP) and co-funded by the health sector, the local authority and SIP. Disadvantaged and vulnerable residents are referred from a variety of agencies. They can participate in a health club providing free access to services focused on reducing stress, stopping smoking, reducing weight and increasing exercise. Health checks are provided, including monitoring CHD risk, a stress level indicator and clinical tests. Service providers include public and private sector agencies. A version of the programme for 3–18 year olds is also running (Junior 'Up for it?').

Specific services aimed at particular health behaviours also offer opportunities to pharmacies[13] – 'Stop Smoking' is one example, as in Box 6.11. As a minimum, pharmacies respond to requests for advice about stopping smoking and can sell nicotine replacement products. Different outlets and staff, including general practices, community pharmacies and others, provide NHS Stop Smoking services. Some PCTs already commission Stop Smoking as an *enhanced* service.

Box 6.11: Stop Smoking: Harrow PCT

Since 2004, the Stop Smoking service in Harrow has been community pharmacy led. Referrals come from dentists, hospitals, district nurses and health visitors, as well as staff in general practices. The service is provided from mosques and schools, and at local employers' premises, as well as the pharmacy.

Community pharmacies have been proposed for weight management services. Box 6.12 describes a community based model for weight management using community development funding, and another private sector model with a stronger medicines element.

Box 6.12: Weight management in community pharmacies

The healthy weight challenge
An independent community pharmacy in Belfast set up the 'Healthy Weight Challenge' in partnership with the Falls Road Women's Centre, funded by community development resources. The pharmacist worked closely with women from the group to design a service that would encourage women to participate and not over-medicalise the problem of weight management. The concept of 'healthy weight' was used instead of words like 'fat' and 'obese'. The service was advertised by posters, leaflets and a local newspaper. Participants met with the pharmacist in the consultation area of the pharmacy for a private discussion about diet and exercise. The pharmacist learnt that causes of excess weight were complex and often socially based. Interventions involved lifestyle, social and health elements. By the end of the pilot period 75 people (73 were women) had participated, of whom 38 were classified as 'overweight' and invited to attend 'healthy weight classes'. Most participants were aged 30–49 years. At follow-up, 24 of the 38 (63%) patients lost weight, 12 had stayed the same weight and two had put on weight.[9]

Boots weight loss programme
A weight loss programme that includes access to orlistat (Xenical) via a private PGD is provided in 100 Boots pharmacies. Registered bodies can issue PGDs for the private supply of prescription-only medicines outside the scope of the NHS. Boots was the first pharmacy to be registered as an independent medical agency by the Healthcare Commission. The weight loss programme is open to adults with a BMI of 30 or more, or 28 or more with other risk factors such as type 2 diabetes or high blood pressure. In an initial 45-minute consultation, the pharmacist measures BMI, blood pressure and blood glucose to check patients' eligibility. Consultations include advice on healthy eating and increasing daily

activity, and free access to a support website and helpline. GPs are informed if their patients are taking part, and patients are referred to them if necessary. Customers pay between £10 and £15 per week and are entitled to discounts on weight loss products and equipment. In one store, over 400 patients joined the scheme and, of those people who were eligible for the scheme, only 3% did not continue into the programme. Just over half of the people who were eligible for the programme were found to have high blood pressure or raised blood glucose levels and were referred to their GPs.

Providing a 'signposting' service

The 'signposting' service provides support by informing patients of other resources and making referrals, where appropriate, to other health care providers, social care providers and support organisations. The local PCT is responsible for providing the pharmacy with a list of relevant resources. The amount of information provided by PCTs and the balance between local and national contacts provided varies between areas. Three PCTs in the Rugby area have jointly produced a signposting resource in the form of a ring binder that has been distributed to pharmacies and general practices. The pharmacy contract encourages recording of signposting: 'When the patient is known to the pharmacy staff, a record of the advice or referral *may* [our emphasis] be made on the patient's pharmacy record, when the pharmacist deems it to be of clinical significance'.[1] Such records will enable the pharmacist to follow up progress with the patient at future visits to the pharmacy. Pharmacists can use the records to monitor and audit signposting, its usefulness and whether it should be augmented or changed.

Some areas have been proactive in their implementation of signposting. The local pharmacy committee (LPC) and the PCT lead for the EPP in Newcastle-under-Lyme PCT developed a concordat whereby pharmacists promoted EPP to patients. The pharmacies stocked leaflets and put them into prescription medicine bags to signpost to local EPP courses. Pharmacists can also signpost people to self care skills training run locally for members of the public, and developed by the WiPP.

Pharmacists can signpost patients to websites with relevant information about their conditions. Box 6.13 contains some useful resources for signposting.

Box 6.13: Resources for signposting

Patient UK

Patient UK (www.patient.co.uk) is a collaboration between the Electronic Medical Information Service (EMIS) and Patient Information Publications (PiP). The website provides non-medical people with good quality information about health and disease. Resources include almost 700 patient information leaflets on health and disease, a directory of almost 2000 patient support organisations and information about medicines. The patient information leaflets and directory of organisations are included in the EMIS clinical system used by GP practices.

> **Directory of Patient Experience (DiPEx)**
> DiPEx (www.dipex.org) brings together patients' experiences, in their own words, on illnesses including cancers, hypertension and epilepsy.
>
> **BestTreatments**
> BestTreatments provides information for patients and, separately, for health professionals on over 80 conditions and surgical procedures.[14] Access is at www.besttreatments.co.uk/btuk/home.html.
>
> **NHS Direct Healthcare guide online**
> The NHS Direct self care guide covers the most common symptoms which people call NHS Direct about for advice. It is available online at www.nhsdirect.nhs.uk.

Making it happen

Actions needed for *essential* services

1 *Support for self care*
   - update protocols/standard operating procedures (SOPs) for medicine sales
   - identify the framework for record keeping and ensure opportunistic interventions are recorded in the pharmacy computer's patient medication record (PMR) if clinically significant
   - ensure mechanisms are in place for referral if required
   - ensure staff are trained to provide advice and support and there is evidence of initial and ongoing training
   - work with local practices to ensure consistency and provide joint support for self care
2 *Promoting healthy lifestyles and public health*
   - establish mechanisms to identify patients for prescription-linked advice
   - establish mechanisms to record advice given
   - write or adapt SOP for prescription-linked advice process
   - identify links to 'signposting' service (e.g. local services for exercise)
   - ensure staff receive training to deliver consistent messages
   - order suitable leaflets
3 *Signposting*
   - write or adapt SOP for service (advised but not compulsory)
   - obtain a compendium of resources from PCT
   - ensure staff are aware of the 'signposting' compendium
   - ensure mechanisms are in place to record referral if clinically significant
   - agree a referral policy with local prescribers
   - identify or design a referral form

Getting organised for promoting and supporting self care as a pharmacy team

Developing your team

Each member of the pharmacy team needs to understand their role and responsibilities in supporting self care.

- Consider nominating a member of staff to lead on self care support.
- Consider using the *essential*, *advanced* and *enhanced* services specifications and identifying which staff members will be involved in each aspect.
- Include the principles of self care, and resources to support it, in training plans for all staff (*see* Tools 10 and 17).
- Encourage staff to look at available NHS self care support resources online and in hard copy.
- Ensure pharmacist locums can provide continuity, knowing your SOPs and ways of working, and that they have relevant accreditation for *advanced* services.
- Work with local practices to ensure consistency and provide joint support for self care.

Table 6.3 can be used to note actions already taken and identify any further actions needed. Box 6.14 contains examples of training resources that can underpin the promotion of self care in pharmacies.

Suggested actions in Table 6.3 for each component of *essential* services are based on those developed by the Pharmaceutical Services Negotiating Committee (PSNC).[15]

Table 6.3: Mapping services, requirements and resources

	SOPs	*Training*	*Records*	*Resources*	*Staff involved*
Self-limiting problems (*essential* service)					
Long term conditions (*essential* service)					
Public health (*essential* service) 1 Campaigns 2 Prescription-linked interventions					
'Signposting' (*essential* service)					

> **Box 6.14:** Training resources to support self care
>
> The NHS Centre for Pharmacy Postgraduate Education provides workshops and open learning including:
> - developing a minor ailments service (open learning pack)
> - minor ailments – supporting self care (workshop)
> - complementary medicines and therapies (open learning pack)
> - smoking cessation (CD ROM)
> - the new contractual framework – clinical effectiveness, audit and record keeping (workshop and open learning pack)
> - practice management: 'Managing Your Resources – people' (workshop)[16]

The National Pharmacy Association offers 'NPA Link Membership' to locum pharmacists who can then access certain NPA resources including education, training and the information department.[17]

Patient and public awareness of new pharmacy services

While patients and the public are supportive of the new community pharmacy contract, general awareness of the changes it is bringing is low. PCTs and pharmacies should work together to raise public awareness. Pharmacists' initial experience of inviting patients to attend a medicines use review, for example, shows that proactive information giving is needed, including use of the booklet highlighted in Box 6.15.

> **Box 6.15:** Resources to inform patients and the public about new services
>
> **Medicines use review**
>
> The Medicines Partnership, supported by the Department of Health, have produced a booklet for patients which explains what a MUR is and enables patients to prepare for their reviews.[18]

Patients also need information about prescription-linked interventions (PLI). These interventions will be opportunistic and triggered by a prescription for treatments for diabetes or CHD. An information leaflet summarising the changes that patients can expect to experience when visiting the pharmacy, and the reasons why, could help to prepare patients. Pharmacists could produce such a leaflet with their PCT.

Quality and audit

The community pharmacy contract has a strong focus on quality.[1] Clinical governance requirements in the *essential* services component of the pharmacy contract are wide ranging. They pose a challenge in developing a culture where clinical governance becomes second nature. Box 6.16 indicates resources that support clinical governance.

> **Box 6.16:** Resources to support clinical governance
>
> **Clinical governance and the new pharmacy contract – just what is required?**[19]
>
> The Royal Pharmaceutical Society of Great Britain (RPSGB) has a series of resources to support community pharmacy audit. Audit templates are available from RPSGB and a selection relevant to self care are included below.
>
> **RPSGB Audit templates relating to self care**
>
> - *Non-prescription medicines – referrals between pharmacist and GP*: an audit of cross-referrals between pharmacists and GPs
> - *Requests for non-prescription medicines*: measures the safety of pharmacy only sales for a certain drug or group of drugs
> - *Responding to symptoms*: suitability of questioning of a customer asking for advice for treating a symptom.
> - *Availability of leaflets*: ensuring that appropriate health information leaflets are available in the pharmacy
> - *Health promotion – smoking cessation campaign*: evaluation of a smoking cessation campaign (part of the 'Ready to go' series)
> - *Health promotion – travel health*: sun awareness campaigns and other travel health issues
> - *Patients' knowledge of the correct use of the oral contraceptive pill*: concerns patients being informed about the correct use of the oral contraceptive pill.
>
> The RPSGB has produced the following resources for interprofessional clinical audits:
>
> - *Improving patient care – a team approach*: guidance about involving community pharmacists in multiprofessional clinical audit. It looks at what can be gained from involving community pharmacists and the main barriers to their involvement
> - *Improving patient care – a team approach*: contains 10 examples of multiprofessional clinical audits involving community pharmacists. These include use of aspirin in secondary prevention of cardiovascular disease, patient's knowledge of emergency contraception, patient compliance in mental health.
>
> The RPSGB also produces guidelines on specific aspects of practice such as that on medicines switched from POM to P (e.g. chloramphenicol eye drops, simvastatin) and on health improvement (e.g. obesity, stopping smoking). All of these resources are freely available on the RSPGB website.[20]

Clinical audits play an important role in the quality of self care-related advice and services provided by a community pharmacy, as in Box 6.17. The contract requires that 'pharmacists and their staff should participate in clinical audit – at least one practice based audit and one PCT determined multidisciplinary audit (to aid the development of team working) each year. The PCT must give reasonable notice to allow the pharmacist to leave the premises to participate in any local meetings relating to the multidisciplinary audit. Both audits must have a clear outcome, which will assist with developing patient care. The two audits should be capable of being completed within five days of pharmacist time'.[1]

> **Box 6.17:** Multidisciplinary clinical audit
>
> Many PCTs, in thinking about multidisciplinary audit, plan to start with a simple audit in the first year to introduce the principle and build local relationships. In many cases the audit is likely to be linked to general medical practice, and while participation in one multidisciplinary audit per year is a compulsory part of the community pharmacy contract there is no requirement for general medical practice to do so. Engaging GPs by finding a common agenda will be an important part of the topic selection process.

Strengthening links in primary care

Pharmacies need to have working links with their PCT, service commissioners, local GP practices, other primary care health professionals, social care and with effective patient and public involvement – as in the examples given in Box 6.18.

Having a good understanding of the local PCT's priorities and of how the GP contract steers the priorities of local GP practices,[5] is important as a basis for targeting particular groups of the public for advice and information, as well as giving opportunities to be commissioned to provide *enhanced* services. Understanding how future commissioning will work under practice based commissioning is essential for community pharmacy.

Communication between community pharmacy and general practice staff will become increasingly important. Multidisciplinary training will offer the chance to build and strengthen links, for example through the training course on self care underpinned by this book.[21]

> **Box 6.18:** Examples of collaborative working between pharmacies and others in primary care
>
> - Stockport's prescribing incentive scheme includes payments for GPs and community pharmacists for holding quarterly joint meetings provided the meeting minutes are submitted to the PCT.
> - Elsewhere, a community pharmacist has been attending his local general practice meeting on a quarterly basis for over a year. He was initially apprehensive about making contact with the practice, but updated them when simvastatin moved from being a prescription only medicine to becoming available OTC. The pharmacist and practice agreed how requests for OTC simvastatin would be dealt with and who would be referred to the practice. Since then, regular contact has continued.
> - Some PCTs have developed a local enhanced service (LES) on self care for their GP practices, for example in Erewash, Southwark and Lambeth PCTs.

Building relationships is more straightforward for community pharmacies that dispense prescriptions for patients from one or two general practices, than for a city centre pharmacy where many general practices are involved. Local workshops to introduce repeat dispensing have helped because pharmacists have met GPs they did not previously know. As repeat dispensing requires clear communication protocols, it has 'kick started' greater collaboration between pharmacies and practices.

Primary care links have been strengthened through the development of local strategies where pharmacy contributes to delivery on key health service targets. Hillingdon LPC and the PCT worked together to develop a community pharmacy strategy (*see* Box 6.19).

Box 6.19: The community pharmacy strategy in Hillingdon PCT

The strategy was created to help the PCT regain financial balance, to offer patients a more versatile choice of treatment options and healthcare service provision and to utilise the skills and accessibility of community pharmacists in Hillingdon. It took into account financial benefit (savings on drugs budget and other budgets):

1　PCT priority (using the LDP and national priorities as guidance)
2　urgent and unmet needs identified from Hillingdon PCT's pharmaceutical needs assessment
3　access to services for patients
4　ease of delivery (taking into account current skills and capacity in community pharmacy and other health care outlets)
5　patient-led demand.

After several group meetings of the pharmacy strategy group (including members of the PCT's medicines management department, the chair and secretary of the LPC and local pharmacists), several areas were identified where pharmacists could make significant advances. These were further developed into potential services that could have a significant impact on patient care, broadly based on five principal areas:

- phlebotomy
- anticoagulation
- respiratory
- weight management
- elderly care.

Potential service specifications were then developed for the identified key areas.

Conclusion

Community pharmacies will extend their involvement and support self care as a result of their new community pharmacy contractual framework. PCTs, general practices and pharmacists should be proactive in ensuring that advice, information and support from the pharmacy are linked to local services and practice. These changes will help to improve the integration of community pharmacy into primary care and to increase recognition of pharmacy's contribution to supporting patients and the public.

References

1. Pharmaceutical Services Negotiating Committee. *New Contract: index and service details.* Aylesbury: PSNC; 2005.
2. The European Society of General Practice/Family Medicine (WONCA). *The European Definition of General Practice/Family Medicine.* Barcelona: WONCA Europe; 2002.
3. Pharmaceutical Services Negotiating Committee. www.psnc.org.uk
4. Department of Health. *Prescribing Guidance.* London: Department of Health; 2003.
5. The General Practitioners Committee/The NHS Confederation. *New GMS Contract. Investing in General Practice.* London: British Medical Association; 2003.
6. Kerins M, Maguire E, Fahey DK et al. Emergency contraception. Has over the counter availability reduced attendance at emergency departments? *Emergency Medicine Journal.* 2004; **21**: 67–8.
7. Anderson C and Blenkinsopp A. Community pharmacy supply of emergency hormonal contraception: a structured literature review of international evidence. *Human Reproduction.* 2006; **21**: 272–84.
8. Modernisation Agency. *Management of Long Term Conditions – what's in it for pharmacists?* London: Department of Health; 2004.
9. Department of Health. *Choosing Health through Pharmacy.* London: Department of Health; 2005.
10. Covey D. *Joint Pharmacy Asthma Project to Launch.* London: Asthma UK; 2005.
11. Modernisation Agency. *Integrating Community Pharmacy into Chronic Disease Management.* London: Department of Health; 2004.
12. Department of Health. *Supporting People with Long Term Conditions – an NHS and social care model to support local innovation and integration.* London: Department of Health; 2005.
13. National Institute for Health and Clinical Excellence. *Helping Smokers to Stop: advice for pharmacists in England.* London: NICE; 2005.
14. www.clinicalevidence.com
15. Pharmaceutical Services Negotiating Committee. *New Contract Workbook.* Aylesbury: PSNC; 2005. www.psnc.org.uk
16. www.cppe.man.ac.uk
17. www.npa.co.uk/departments/membership.html
18. Medicines Partnership. www.medicines-partnership.org/our-publications
19. www.cgsupport.nhs.uk/Primary_Care/Pharmacy/What_is_Required-ques-.asp
20. Royal Pharmaceutical Society of Great Britain. www.rpsgb.org
21. Working in Partnership Programme. www.wipp.nhs.uk

7

Seeing self care from the patient's perspective

Ruth Chambers, Health First and Matthew Critchlow

This chapter considers the patient's perspective. It gives patients' views about the nature of support for self care that is currently available in the NHS. Then it discusses what we can do to improve the range of self care resources available and the manner in which we promote and support self care.

Many people already practise self care to a greater or lesser extent, as the report in Box 7.1 of focus group discussions demonstrates.[1] Patients participating considered that there were four main issues that require self care or self management:

- medical issues (such as drug side-effects and changing diet)
- emotional and psychological issues (such as isolation and low mood)
- making lifestyle changes
- gaining a thorough understanding of their disease, which can enhance motivation to self care and help to guide decision making about alternative actions.[1]

Box 7.1: Patients' reported self care

In a series of two focus groups organised by Health First the 18 patients who discussed self care emphasised the importance of being assertive with the doctors and nurses looking after them to obtain optimal advice and treatment for their conditions.[1] Establishing a relationship of trust between health professional and patient was thought to be key.

Self managing the emotional and psychological consequences of a long term health condition was seen as key, as mental wellbeing impacts on an individual's motivation to self care. Patients taking part appeared to have received minimal guidance from health professionals about the emotional and psychological side of coping with their illness, relying on friends, family and other patients through informal self help and peer-to-peer support instead. Some patients had benefited from 'positive thinking' (e.g. cognitive techniques) to take care of their emotional issues.

Many of those participating reported using complementary therapies (e.g. massage, acupuncture, herbal medicine) when taking care of their long term conditions.

Patients' definition of self care

Patients' views of self care are mainly concerned with the practical tasks or behaviours involved, including issues such as taking medication and exercising, and gaining knowledge of the disease. Some of the patients participating in the focus group discussions (see Box 7.1) had a broader understanding of self care (see Box 7.2). Those who had been through the Expert Patients Programme (EPP) mentioned a more individualised approach to self care 'fine tuning what works for you', reflecting the problem solving approach included in EPP training (see Box 7.7 also). Some appreciated the beliefs and attitudes associated with self caring such as 'taking responsibility' and 'making one's own decisions'.

Box 7.2: Definition of self care by patients themselves

Practical elements

- Taking care of your own health e.g. taking medication, changing diet, exercising
- Doing your own research and gaining knowledge of the disease
- Finding alternatives and fine tuning what works for you
- Entertaining your mind
- Relating to others with a similar condition

Attitudes/beliefs

- Taking responsibility and making your own decisions
- Having confidence[1]

Health professionals could consider expanding their definition of self care to include the beliefs associated with self caring behaviour.

How are patients self managing or self caring at present?

Managing treatment

Patients' self-initiated approaches to treatment can include the use of complementary therapies. A patient can sometimes mistakenly make inappropriate management decisions, such as stopping conventional medicine due to side-effects, in favour of unproven alternatives such as herbal medicine for the treatment of conditions such as hypertension. Complementary approaches play a significant role in many patients' self care. Patients need reliable information and advice about complementary treatments and how to select appropriate treatments (e.g. which questions to ask when exploring and making an assessment of alternatives).

Minor ailments like sore throat are self limiting and can be alleviated or resolved with OTC treatments or other self care approaches (see Chapter 6).

Managing emotional/psychological issues

The emphasis for patients should be on thinking positively, accepting their condition and building motivation and self-confidence. There is clearly a link between someone's ability to manage emotional and psychological issues and their motivation to self care. Coping with emotional issues may be a key first hurdle in successfully self caring for their health condition. Patients will gain support from a variety of sources (*see* Box 7.3), including their religious faith. Learning and practising cognitive techniques such as positive thinking and re-framing (i.e. turning negatives into positives) can help. Effective guidance from health professionals in dealing with issues such as denial, bereavement and low mood will help too.

Box 7.3: Sources of health information that may influence help-seeking behaviour[2]

- Family, friends, work colleagues, acquaintances
- Community leaders, local people recognised as sources of health-related advice
- Self help groups, self care support networks and community and voluntary organisations
- Consumer health information and advice services
- Telephone helplines and high street and hospital information points
- Health food retailers
- High street pharmacists
- Health care providers outside the NHS (e.g. acupuncturists, chiropractors)
- Healthcare providers within the NHS (e.g. dentists, doctors, nurses)
- Individuals associated with healthcare providers (e.g. relatives and friends of health professionals)
- Pharmaceutical companies
- The media (newspapers, soap operas, dramas etc)

Making lifestyle changes

Patients may take up various forms of exercise, change to a better diet or limit the amount of alcohol they drink to within recommended levels. They can draw on a variety of resources that can help them change.

Professional bodies, local communities, general practices and others offer a whole range of activities to encourage people to make and sustain lifestyle changes (*see* Box 7.4).

Box 7.4: Examples of resources and support for improved lifestyles for patients and the public

- Stafford Borough Council offers free led walks in its 'Walk Wise' initiative – half hour walks that anyone can join.[3]

- Pharmacists offer structured stop smoking programmes.
- The Chartered Society of Physiotherapy has produced *The Lazy Exercise Guide for Busy People* that indicates how physical activity can be incorporated into someone's everyday life.[4]
- Local NHS trusts in association with Dr Foster[5] publish a free magazine for 'lads in their twenties' and a similar version for young women. The *FIT* magazine has general information on lifestyle habits – sex, illicit drugs, smoking, alcohol consumption, etc, with local information. The magazine has a similar look to commercially available ones which also contain pertinent articles about improving health and lifestyle – such as *Men's Health*.
- The Arthritis Research Campaign (and similarly other disease specific organisations) produce a variety of booklets and other types of information that encourage a healthy lifestyle for arthritis sufferers and better managing their disease.[6]
- Cancer Research UK publishes material designed to help people halve their risks of cancer through stopping smoking, staying in shape, eating and drinking healthily, avoiding sunburn and attending recommended health screening.[7]
- MIND produces a range of self care booklets for patients to improve their mental wellbeing including such topics as: *The MIND Guide to Relaxation, How to Cope as a Carer, How to Assert Yourself, How to Look after Yourself.*[8]

Gaining knowledge of their disease

Knowing about their disease or ill health should help patients in taking care of themselves. The internet is one of the more commonly used sources of information, although books, self care support networks and alternative therapists all contribute.

At present, people are exposed to many competing and often inconsistent messages from diverse sources. Patients need guidance on appropriate and easily accessible sources of information from the internet where the quality and reliability of information can be variable (*see* p. 107).

Various organisations produce materials to aid people's quest for knowledge about their disease (*see* Box 7.5 for examples).

Box 7.5: Examples of organisations that encourage people to learn more about their disease and treatment options
- Allergy UK has developed a patient self assessment checklist for asthma.
- The Consumer Health Information Centre (CHIC) produces quick reference guides for a general readership, e.g. a guide to allergies with a searchable online database of products to treat minor ailments.[9]
- Diabetes UK.[10]
- The Developing Patient Partnerships (DPP) produce a range of materials to support their regular campaigns in association with PCTs – these covered

minor ailments, sexual health, obesity, mental health in 2005 – enabling patients and the public to take care of their own health.[11] Some materials are produced in association with other bodies such as the Royal Pharmaceutical Society, National Pharmacy Association and CHIC, e.g. a self-help guide to childhood ailments.
- Family Doctor Books are published in association with the British Medical Association. They are available for purchase through pharmacies or from the website.[12]
- Nurse practitioners, diabetes nurse specialists and other specialist nurses, in particular, provide useful, in-depth, information on the disease as well as practical advice on self care in an interactive style.[1] Patients value health professionals taking time to provide detailed information that is relevant to them, and not taking for granted what they may or may not already understand about their condition. The focus should be on providing disease information that is tailored to the individual, encompassing both detailed background on the condition and self care skills (e.g. self-monitoring and managing diet).

What could patients do to achieve a higher level of self care and increase their 'response-ability'?

Know more about their disease

Patients need to gain a thorough and realistic understanding of their disease and its progression, to find out about the actions they can take in relation to self care (*see* the various elements listed in Box 7.6).

Box 7.6: Gaining knowledge of the disease
- Gain a realistic understanding of the condition
- Understand the progression of their disease
- Learn how to look after themselves
- Gain knowledge for themselves (including doing research on the internet)
- Know about availability of resources, e.g. disabled parking stickers, self care support networks and other groups

Patients who are better informed about their condition tend to be more motivated to self care. If patients have a good understanding of the severity of their condition, the long term implications (partly based on knowledge of family history and other individual risk factors), the consequences of not caring, and their ability to recover, they are more likely to look after themselves.

Patients with a higher level of education appear to be more motivated to self care, which may be linked to their tendency to be better informed about their condition.

Patients in these groups often have greater access to information and have greater confidence in asking questions and making decisions about their health.

The *Expert Patients Programme* (EPP) aims to improve the quality of life of a person with a long term condition, by developing their generic knowledge and skills, confidence and motivation to take more effective control over their life and illness.[13,14] The six week course is available to anyone with a long term condition. It may be delivered by trained volunteers and paid trainers through PCTs or some voluntary organisations licensed to deliver the course. Many of those participating in such programmes report being in better health, coping better with fatigue, feeling less limited in what they can do and being less dependent on hospital care. Box 7.7 describes the aims of the programme for individuals taking part.

Box 7.7: The aims of the Expert Patients Programme

EPP helps people to:

- prevent conditions from becoming worse
- make comfortable comparisons with each other
- provide somewhere to voice an unmet need
- see that their symptoms are 'normal'
- recognise and act on their symptoms
- make more effective use of medicines and treatments
- understand the implications of professional advice
- access social and other services including transport
- manage work and access the resources of the employment services
- access chosen leisure activities
- develop strategies to deal with the psychological effects of illness.[13-15]

Most PCTs have a self care support co-ordinator who recruits and trains people living with long term conditions to deliver the lay-led courses as volunteer tutors. The co-ordinator monitors the quality of the paid trainers and volunteer tutors. They also manage and facilitate EPP courses, promote the course to potential referrers from the health, social care and voluntary sectors, and recruit patients and carers to undertake the programme.[13,14] PCTs need to try harder to improve their engagement with community and voluntary groups and patients from disadvantaged and ethnic minority groups, to encourage people to attend the EPP which is available in the NHS throughout England (*see* Box 7.8).[15-17] An online internet version of EPP is being piloted.

Box 7.8: A review of the implementation of the EPP pilot

A recent review of the EPP programme found that it appealed strongly to white middle class female patients, compared to those living in deprived areas.[15] There were opposing views about the value of the course being generic or adapted to individual long term conditions. Some trusts, such as Burnley/Pendle/

Seeing self care from the patient's perspective

Rossendale PCT, have developed a related programme specific to diabetes. The outcome most valued was the social support generated by sharing experiences, practical exchange of ideas and reduction in social isolation. The mutually supportive networks persist after the six week course in many areas, but more work needs to be done to ensure that the networks are sustained elsewhere.

At the beginning of the pilot, the vast majority of health professionals in primary care were not engaged by the EPP – but now there is greater awareness of EPP as it is mainstreamed.

Internal monitoring of the pilot phase has described a significant decrease in use of some healthcare services after an EPP course: 7% decrease in GP consultations, 10% decrease in outpatient visits, and 16% fewer A&E attendances. Many participants noted improvements in their symptoms: 37% reported less intense pain, 43% a decrease in tiredness, 39% a lessening of depression, and 33% reduction in breathlessness.[18]

Access reliable information about possible symptoms and signs of illness and take action accordingly

NHS Direct provides 24-hour healthcare information and advice for the general population at an affordable cost (*see* Box 7.9). By September 2005, NHS Direct had taken 29 million telephone calls.[19] Patients have access to health advice by phone, day or night. NHS Direct provides a symptomatic clinical assessment. Users can either self care or access NHS services for treatment in a timely way. NHS Direct operates an online resource[20] as well as an interactive digital TV platform and the well known telephone helpline (0845 4647). The telephone service can handle enquiries in a variety of languages. The online service receives 12 to 15 million visits a year which is likely to increase. The NHS Direct interactive TV service is also growing, with more than 30% of households having access to digital satellite TV now. The paper version of the NHS self care guide is available in large print and Braille.[21] The website also has an extended version of this e-NHS Direct guide with answers to frequently asked health questions.[20] People can send their own enquiry to the website too or search for their nearest doctor, dentist or pharmacist.

Box 7.9: Costs of NHS Direct

The NHS Direct service costs around £2.40 per person per year in England (at 2005 prices) to run.[19] This covers the telephone helpline, website and digital TV resources and the self care guide.

Other organisations such as Developing Patient Partnerships produce literature to guide people as to what to do when unwell, and signpost relevant NHS services.[11]

The Association of the British Pharmaceutical Industry (ABPI) produces an updated guide and directory on health and medicines – helping patients ask the right questions of health professionals and rating the quality of information obtained or given.[22]

Other countries have developed similar self care support resources – British Columbia has a local version of the *Healthwise* handbook which includes basic guidelines on how to recognise and cope with more than 200 common health problems.[23] It gives information on prevention, home treatment, emergencies, when to call a health professional and healthy lifestyle choices. There is an associated 24-hour nurse line that can answer questions about symptoms, health concerns, and recommend courses of action etc, and an online resource.[24]

Work effectively with health professionals

Core ingredients for patients and health professionals to work together effectively are actively seeking advice, feedback and making decisions together. To do this the health professional needs to gain the trust of the patient.

Part of making decisions together is developing self care plans. Self care and self management plans do not seem to be widely used – common examples are restricted to diabetes and asthma. These plans could include advice on the management of emotional and psychological issues as well as self-administration of drugs and symptom or blood monitoring.

Patients should not be too afraid or shy to ask for help or advice from the health professionals treating them. Give patients plenty of opportunities for discussion, so that they do not feel rushed in their consultation with insufficient time to ask the questions they want to pose. The NHS may have to help patients develop skills in assertiveness if they want to increase their knowledge and skills in self care, to develop their questioning skills and expressions of wants, needs and ideas in appropriate ways.

Elderly patients are less likely to self care because they are often less well informed about their condition, tend to be more physically impaired and are more likely to take a passive approach to their healthcare, i.e. 'Dr knows best'. Elderly, less well educated and non-Westernised people are less likely to manage their own minor ailments and continue to consult their GP instead.[25] Younger patients are generally more likely to take an active role in their care, but can also be unwilling to conform to advice.

Pharmacists are ideally placed to advise people about their health and provide preventive advice as well as treatment. Community pharmacists see as many as six million people a day in the UK, both well and ill people.[26] Their new contract promotes healthy lifestyles – they could introduce services such as blood pressure testing, weight measurement, carbon monoxide breath analysis for smokers and health 'MOTs'.[27]

Teachers are another group of professionals with an impact on people's personal health decisions. 'Making Sense of Health' is developing teachers' professional skills in health education of young people – another scheme within the WPP.

Contact self-help and peer-to-peer self care support networks and groups

Self-help groups and self care support networks play an important role in supporting self care amongst certain types of patients and can provide valuable information for health professionals in understanding barriers to self care (*see* p. 24). Confidentiality issues may have to be overcome in peer-to-peer support groups if people raise them.

Boost their personal motivation

Box 7.10 summarises the main factors that determine the extent to which people provide self care for themselves. Patients with higher levels of motivation to self care may be more internally motivated, showing greater determination to gain control of their health, and accept responsibility in looking after their own health.[28] People with higher motivation tend to perceive the disease as something that they can gain control over and live with. In contrast, patients with lower motivation for self caring, take less responsibility for looking after their own health and adopt the attitude that it is the responsibility of others, i.e. the care system or health professionals, to look after them. In extreme cases, patients with low motivation may experience a high degree of helplessness faced with a health problem – such as 'I'm going to have a poor quality of life; there's nothing that I can do about the situation'.

These differences in motivation may be linked to their personality type. Those patients with an inherently positive outlook (optimists) show greater motivation to self care. Those with a more negative outlook (more pessimistic) are less motivated to self care.

Box 7.10: Determinants of a person's level of self care
- Internal or external motivation
- Determination or will to take control of health
- Habits, myths and beliefs
- Patient's perception of the disease and quality of life
- Personality – positive versus negative outlook

If symptoms of their condition are more obvious and tangible, they act as a constant reminder of the condition, thereby helping to motivate a patient to self care. Those patients with less obvious symptoms (e.g. hypertension) tend to be less motivated to self care. People with low mood and depression in response to developing a long term condition may be apathetic and lack a desire to self care.

Family members can help to motivate patients to self care. However, some carers take too much responsibility upon themselves and do not encourage the patient to self care independently. People with diabetes may be actively 'managed' by their partners in relation to their diet, blood monitoring, etc. This causes particular problems if the partner or carer dies or has to go away and patients are not able to manage on their own.

Attitudes towards health, disease and self care vary according to cultural background. This can have a negative impact on levels of self care if individuals are less engaged with health professionals. *See* the example given in Box 7.11.

Box 7.11: Example of the impact of culture on perception of health and likelihood to self care

A GP talked about some of her West African patients who do not view high blood pressure as a health problem and see obesity as a sign of wealth and health, rather than an adverse factor in relation to their health. Motivation to self manage these conditions is, therefore, low. Furthermore, certain patients from this population receive treatment from others such as elders, church leaders, spiritual healers and herbalists.[1]

Understand physical constraints and personal circumstances

Some stroke patients, for example, have physical or cognitive impairments that make self care difficult. Other patients may have caring responsibilities (i.e. children or other dependants), that restrict their ability to undertake self care for themselves.

Improve health at work

The work place is a setting for health promotion and self care.[29] Work is important to maintain a person's health and wellbeing, as well as earning an income.[30] The national strategy aims to help people avoid work-related problems as well as take care of minor health problems at work with access to appropriate treatment – such as for sprains and muscular strains.

The Chartered Society of Physiotherapy offers advice and treatment for a range of health problems that might impinge on people's fitness for work. They advise people to undertake certain exercises every hour or so to reduce their risk of developing work-related aches and pains, to avoid sitting for too long, and to get up and stretch every 20 minutes or so.[31]

Research by the Developing Patient Partnerships (DPP) organisation has found that if employees had more information from their employer about taking care of common ailments they would be less likely to take time off work.[32] Resources include campaign materials, health bulletins, patient education of all sorts and health toolkits – for PCTs and practices too. DPP provide a health at work service comprising regular campaigns (e.g. beating back pain), health bulletins and health toolkits with personal health folders for employees, and advice and support for employers in promoting occupational health and managing sickness absence.[33]

Other community initiatives to get people back to work, as in Box 7.12, can further boost health and self care opportunities.

> **Box 7.12:** Examples of projects helping unemployed people back to work
>
> **Learning and Employment Action Package (LEAP)**
> The LEAP project is headed by Connexions Staffordshire. It helps people gain employment through a programme of in-depth, continuous support and job mentoring. The programme is free and confidential and supports people in the early stages of their employment. LEAP is for anyone who is unemployed, between 16 and 65 years of age and who is not claiming Job Seeker's Allowance. It specifically targets lone parents, ex-offenders, the long term unemployed, people with disabilities and those from minority ethnic groups. A team of job

> mentors meets with clients as often as they require and at convenient locations for them.
>
> **Next Moves**
> Next Moves offers a range of specialist services and activities to motivate and support individuals as soon as they become unemployed. Connexions adult advisers work with adults when they register with Jobcentre Plus. Participants can sign up for up to 16 hours per week for a maximum of 13 weeks. Participants have free access to newspapers, postage, telephone and the internet to search for jobs. Sixty per cent of those entering the programme are expected to move quickly into employment.

Understand more about complementary health care

Many people buy complementary and alternative medicine (CAM) therapies – around 10% of the population visit a CAM practitioner in any year. So any self care approach should take into account the thinking and practice of complementary health care. Health professionals need to know that people are taking or using complementary therapies that might interact with prescribed medicines or cause adverse effects.

About half of all general practices in England offer patients access to complementary therapies.[34] The extent to which these can be integrated into conventional primary care provision is a balancing act between patients' expectations and needs, and accepted standards of medical and scientific principles of practice.[35]

Who provides complementary therapies?

Some complementary practitioners are practising health professionals such as doctors, physiotherapists or nurses who are state registered with their own professional organisations. Others such as osteopaths and chiropractors are registered with their own statutory bodies. Most complementary practitioners have completed further education in their discipline. Their knowledge and skills mainly come from training based on what has been passed down by tradition rather than proven by scientific evidence.

Many conventional health professionals practise in the typically holistic manner of complementary therapists too (*see* Figure 5.1, p. 54). Scientific, artistic and spiritual insights need to be applied together to restore health. Holistic practitioners believe that illness provides opportunities for positive change as you reflect on your circumstances, and create a better balance to your life. People opt for complementary therapies because they are 'low tech', or because their symptoms are persisting, or as a result of real or perceived adverse effects from conventional treatments.[36]

The evidence for complementary therapies

There is not much research evidence on how many of the alternative therapies are effective for exactly what conditions. The Cochrane Collaboration has completed 145 reviews of randomised controlled trials of complementary and alternative therapies:

one-third showed a positive or possibly positive effect, and in over half there was insufficient evidence to make a judgement.[37] Just because acupuncture is proven to be effective for low back pain, does not necessarily mean that it is effective for headaches. For many people it is the placebo effect, the fact that they are taking a treatment, that makes them think the treatment is working. If someone listens to them with interest and uses their hands to massage or treat them, they are likely to leave that consultation feeling better.

Some publications and sources of reference promote complementary healthcare to people as part of a general self care approach, so that they are informed about what a treatment entails, likely benefits or possible risks and costs.[38] The cost effectiveness of complementary treatments to the NHS is still uncertain. A systematic review of cost effectiveness included five research studies; complementary treatments represented an additional cost to usual care in four of the five studies.[39]

References

1 Critchlow M. *Enabling Self Care. Report on focus groups of patients with long term conditions, and healthcare professionals in Southwark and Lambeth PCTs.* London: Health First; 2005.

2 Rogers A, Entwistle V and Pencheon D. A patient led NHS: managing demand at the interface between lay and primary care. *British Medical Journal.* 1998; **316:** 1816–19.

3 www.staffordbc.gov.uk/la21

4 www.csp.org.uk

5 www.drfoster.co.uk

6 www.arc.org.uk

7 www.reducetherisk.org.uk

8 www.mind.org.uk/index.htm

9 www.chic.org.uk

10 www.diabetes.org.uk

11 www.dpp.org.uk

12 www.familydoctor.co.uk

13 Long-term Medical Conditions Alliance (LMCA). *Supporting Expert Patients. How to develop lay led self-management programmes for patients with long-term medical conditions.* London: LMCA; 2001.

14 Department of Health. *Expert Patients Programme Update.* Issue 13. August 2005. www.expertpatients.nhs.uk

15 Rogers A, Bower P, Kennedy A et al. *How has the EPP been Delivered and Accepted in the NHS during the Pilot Phase?* Manchester: National Primary Care Research and Development Centre; 2005.

16 Griffiths C, Motlih J, Azad A et al. Randomised controlled trial of a lay-led self-management programme for Bangladeshi patients with chronic disease. *British Journal of General Practice.* 2005; **55:** 831–7.

17 Cooper J, Thompson J. *Stepping Stones to Success.* Beckenham: Department of Health; 2005.

18 Donaldson L. *Mainstreaming the Expert Patients Programme (EPP)*. Gateway approval 4559. London: Department of Health; 2005.

19 Sadler M. NHS Direct – let the force for patients be with you. *BMJ Careers*. 2005; **10 September:** 111.

20 www.nhsdirect.nhs.uk

21 Banks I. *The NHS Direct Healthcare Guide*. Oxford: Radcliffe Medical Press; 2000.

22 www.askaboutmedicines.org

23 www.healthwise.org

24 www.bchealthguide.org

25 Cardol M, Schellevis FG, Spreeuwenberg P et al. Changes in patients' attitudes towards the management of minor ailments. *British Journal of General Practice*. 2005; **55:** 516–21.

26 McRobbie H and McEwen A. *Helping Smokers to Stop: advice for pharmacists in England*. London: National Institute for Health and Clinical Excellence (NICE), Royal Pharmaceutical Society, PharmacyHealthLink; 2005.

27 National Pharmaceutical Association (NPA). *Pharmacy Contract Service Specification 4 – promotion of healthy lifestyles (public health)*. St Albans: NPA; 2005. www.npa.co.uk

28 McLean J and Pietroni P. Self care – who does best? *Social Science and Medicine*. 1990; **30:** 591–6.

29 Department of Health. *Choosing a Better Diet: a food and health action plan*. London: Department of Health; 2005.

30 Department of Health. *Health, Work and Well-being – caring for our future: a strategy for the health and well-being of working age people*. London: Department of Health; 2005.

31 Chartered Society of Physiotherapy. *Fit to Work*. London: Chartered Society of Physiotherapy; 2005. www.csp.org.uk

32 Developing Patient Partnerships. *Health at Work: workplace health education*. London: DPP; 2005.

33 www.dpphealthatwork.org.uk

34 Thomas KJ, Coleman P and Nicholl JP. Trends in access to complementary or alternative medicines via primary care in England: 1995–2001. Results from a national survey. *Family Practice*. 2003; **20:** 575–7.

35 Frenkel MA and Borkan JM. An approach for integrating complementary–alternative medicine into primary care. *Family Practice*. 2003; **20:** 324–32.

36 Thompson T and Feder G. Complementary therapies and the NHS. *British Medical Journal*. 2005; **331:** 856–7.

37 Manheimer E, Berman B, Dubnick H et al. Cochrane Reviews of Complementary and Alternative Therapy: evaluating the strength of the evidence. 2004. www.cochrane.org/colloquia/abstracts/ottawa/P-094.htm

38 Pinder M, Pedro L, Theodorou G et al. *Complementary Healthcare: a guide for patients*. London: The Prince of Wales's Foundation for Integrated Health; 2005. www.fihealth.org.uk

39 Canter P, Thompson Coon J and Ernst E. Cost effectiveness of complementary treatments in the United Kingdom: systematic review. *British Medical Journal*. 2005; **331:** 880–1.

8
Managing change – moving to a self care culture
Ruth Chambers and Gill Wakley

We need to change our behaviour as an individual health professional or a practice or PCT organisation, if we are to genuinely provide support for self care and enable patients and members of the public to change to self caring behaviour too. So this chapter emphasises how you can make and sustain that change.

The process of change

Look at the flow chart in Figure 8.1 about how people usually react to change. You start off by being taken by surprise about a change, even if you anticipate it. Promoting a culture of self care support across general practices and pharmacies would be a change for most primary care practitioners and teams. You tend to move from the shock of being expected to change to pretending it is not going to happen.

After the denial phase in the change process, you move on to find somebody to blame for what has happened – blaming the messengers who announce the change. After the blame comes self-blame (e.g. 'I'm no good at promoting self care').

Part of the next stage, the bargaining, is negotiating that if you do it *this* way you are going to be able to do *that*. Eventually you arrive at the resolution phase where you have accepted the change.

When change is imposed by others you are very much more resistant, so you move more slowly. If the effect of the change is serious, your feelings about it will be stronger and you will spend longer in the phases of denial, blame and self-blame.[1]

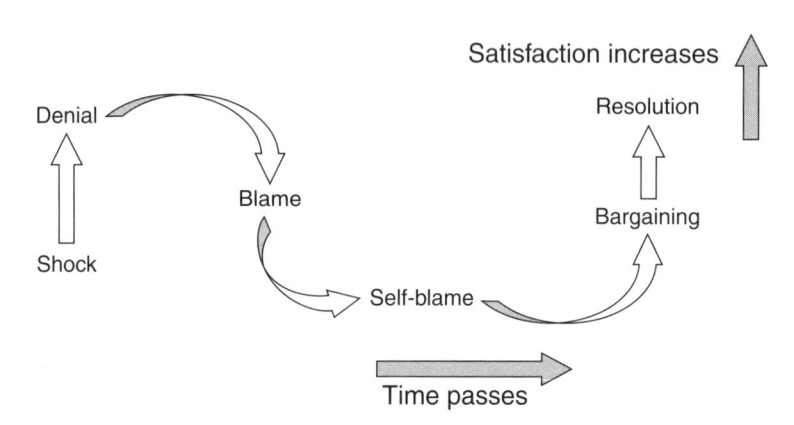

Figure 8.1: Stages in the response to change.

You need to identify clearly the causes for dissatisfaction with the present situation (that is, too little self care by patients), and then have a clear idea of where to head. Map out how to reach that target. Find the way in staged steps to measure your progress towards the target.

People play roles in response to change:[2]

- *the rebel*: 'I don't see why I should'
- *the victim*: 'I suppose you will make me, but I will drag my feet'
- *the oppressor*: 'you all have to do it'
- *the rescuer*: 'I will save you all from this terrible change'.

There is a dearth of evidence about how to secure change in clinical behaviour. There are plenty of worthy books and articles on ways of making and managing change, and much is known about the effects of change on an organisation and workforce. The gaps between theory and practice and the general lack of application of research into clinical practice are well recognised.

Managing change within the PCT or practice

To bring about change and get evidence about the effectiveness of self care into practice:[3]

- consider what individual beliefs, attitudes and knowledge influence professionals' and managers' behaviour
- be aware of important influences in the organisational, economic and community environments of practitioners
- identify factors likely to influence the proposed change
- plan appropriate interventions: multi-faceted interventions developed as an integrated resource targeting different barriers to change are more likely to be effective than single interventions
- interventions are targeted at overcoming potential barriers
- keep people informed by describing the evidence and need for change, in words and ways they can comprehend
- motivate people to tackle the change – show why the change is necessary and important, who else supports the change, how problems associated with the proposed change can be solved
- provide adequate resources to underpin the change of practice – such as people with the right level of knowledge and skills
- incorporate monitoring and evaluation of the change from the planning stage and throughout the activity
- implement the change and find ways to maintain and reinforce the new practices e.g. reminder systems, educational programmes
- disseminate information about the change in ways that are appropriate to the nature and setting of the participants.

The nature of resistance to change will be specific to any particular situation.

Why people do not change

Resistance is a natural, universal, inevitable human response to a change that someone else thinks is a good idea, and resisting change or improvement does not make someone bad or narrow-minded. We have all done it and our response will be one of three things: fight, flight or freeze.

There are lots of reasons why people may be hesitant about changing the way they do things. These may include:

- having a poor appreciation of the need to change or considering the need to change to be secondary to other issues
- having a poor understanding of the proposed solutions or considering the solution to be inappropriate
- disagreeing how the change should be implemented
- embarrassment about admitting that what they are doing could be improved
- lacking trust in a person or the organisation, as they believe it has failed to successfully implement change in the past
- anticipating a lack of resources.

People underestimate the barriers and hurdles to be overcome before change will be made and sustained. Barriers may be:

- lack of perception of relevance
- lack of resources
- short term outlook
- conflicting priorities
- difficulty in measuring outcomes
- lack of necessary skills
- no history of multidisciplinary working
- limitations of the research evidence on effectiveness
- perverse incentives
- intensity of contribution required.

Sometimes the problem arises from a malfunctioning organisation. If so, you need to implement a well thought out and substantial plan to overhaul your PCT or practice and remedy them.

Encouragement to change

Think about four levels of change:[4]

1. do you need to do something new?
2. should you do things differently – change a system or process?
3. should you do something different – change the purpose?
4. do you need to stop doing something – does the service or organisation need to exist at all?

Organisations are like weather systems, constantly changing and shifting. If you change one thing, it affects many others. The environment constantly alters so the outside influences need constant monitoring. Strategies such as yours to establish a new culture of self care must be flexible. People have to be supported in coping with the constant change. Remember to involve them from the outset, keep them informed and part of the change process. Give them time to grieve for the past ways of working and time for criticism and interchange of ideas. Imposing change on your PCT or practice team will breed resentment and resistance to your hopes for their promoting and supporting self care.

Making the transition to supporting self care

Change happens all the time. So establishing a new culture of promoting and supporting self care within your PCT, practice or across your practice team, is just one more challenge for your change management skills. The transition will occur more smoothly by:

- deciding what needs to be changed through gathering evidence about self care
- sharing the responsibility for identifying the problems involved and finding the solutions so that everyone feels part of the process (ownership)
- building in plenty of time to discuss the planned changes so that everyone feels that they have had a chance to put his/her points of view
- making the changes in small steps
- giving plenty of support to everyone in the team, and monitoring progress
- giving feedback so that everyone knows how the changes are progressing and what their part in them means to the whole
- celebrating completion of milestones in your action plan and continuing monitoring to prevent backsliding!

Getting there

People react better if they have a direction of travel. Remember to KISS (keep it simple and short), and pick two or three targets that mark the evolution of your new culture of self care, to focus on – as in Figures 3.1 (*see* p. 33) and 4.1 (*see* p. 44). If you set up too many targets, you will not finish any, and everyone will become discouraged.

Help everyone to understand the current issues and why the change to a culture of self care is necessary and will improve healthcare overall. Identify who is likely to lose what. Some health professionals may perceive they will lose status and power if patients are enabled to care more readily for themselves.

References

1 Upton T and Brooks B. *Managing Change*. Buckingham: Open University Press; 1995.
2 Riley J. *Helping Doctors Who Manage*. London: King's Fund Publishing; 1998.
3 NHS Centre for Reviews and Dissemination. *Getting Evidence into Practice*. Effective Health Care Bulletin 5(1). London: Royal Society of Medicine Press; 1999.
4 Prochaska J, DiClemente C and Norcross J. In search of how people change. *American Psychologist*. 1992; **47:** 1102–14.

9

Completing the cycle: evaluation
Ruth Chambers

It is all very well planning development or setting up a new service, such as extending your range and activity in supporting self care. But is the outcome what you planned for, and are the developments sustained? This chapter suggests how you might monitor or evaluate that your PCT or practice team now promote and support self care for patients and the public as you set out to do.

Evaluation and monitoring are essential components of any programme or service. Incorporate these into any plan to establish a culture of self care or support self care, from the beginning. Time and effort spent on evaluation should be in proportion to the activity that is being evaluated. Keep it as simple as possible and avoid wasting resources on unnecessarily bureaucratic evaluation.

Evaluation sets out measurable targets and timescales that are realistic for the particular context and problems of the population group you are monitoring and auditing. Agree on short, medium and longer term outcomes with all the 'stakeholders' in the PCT and/or practice, before the evaluation begins.[1] There are always risks that other factors may crop up that are not under your control and that the outcomes you originally expected if your initiative worked well, are no longer viable or possible.

Use an approach that is appropriate and relevant to your patients or local population:

- agree what criteria you will use for the outcome of the evaluation, e.g. that you measure what you set out to measure
- invite external review either from an independent person (e.g. the PCT facilitator) or by comparing what you have done against external standards (e.g. what another PCT or practice that is known for its self care work has done)
- assess how well you have done in one area. You might include one or more of: activity, personnel, provision of service, organisational structure or objectives, in your evaluation. You might focus on self care support in relation to particular health topics like sore throat, back pain, asthma or cough.

What to evaluate[2]

You might assess any or every aspect of your strategy and plans for supporting self care and how they were put into practice. Here are some ideas you could use for evaluation – most of them are challenging:

- everyone participated in the actual initiative, by measuring their performance

Completing the cycle: evaluation   119

- the objectives of the action plan to promote and support self care were well phrased, simple, measurable, achievable, realistic and timely
- everyone supported and adhered to any changes within the action plan
- the proposed strategy for self care support and associated action plan were implemented
- training needs that were identified were addressed appropriately
- the way that self care was promoted and supported justified the effort and cost
- there was good leadership of the self care support strategy and action plan throughout the PCT and/or practice team
- progress achieved in promoting and supporting self care was conveyed to everyone affected and results discussed
- there was an emphasis on teamworking and support
- the PCT/practice culture and environment were conducive to supporting self care
- the quality of patient care was improved; health and wellbeing was improved.

Design the evaluation

You might focus your evaluation on:

1. what actually happened – such as the content of self care support interventions
2. how it worked out – how well the self care support interventions were put into practice; how well the different components were integrated
3. the outcome – what you achieved as a result of your self care support interventions.

You might evaluate the 'what', 'how' and 'outcome' of your various self care support programme, or just one of these, such as the 'how' only. Evaluating the outcome, and what you achieved or the changes made to the service you provide to patients as a result, will be more challenging to evaluate than the 'what' and the 'how' aspects.

The plan

- Specify exactly what you are evaluating. Set priorities against what you need to achieve and the time and resources available. Obtain agreement from the PCT/practice or pharmacy team on the nature and scope of the evaluation.
- Describe the expected impact of the programme or activity and who will be affected.
- Define the criteria of success – these might relate to the what, how or outcome (*see above*).
- Identify the information required to demonstrate what the team achieved; e.g. observation, audit, prospective recording by staff or survey of patients receiving self care support.
- Determine what everyone involved in the evaluation will do by what time (*see Tool 7*).

If you are considering the quality of self care support with which a patient is being provided you should question whether it:

- was available – to all patients on an impartial basis (whatever their gender, age, social class, ethnicity, religion, postcode of their residence)

Table 9.1: Criteria for evaluation by PCTs of the extent to which self care is promoted and supported

Aspect of self care	What is it about?	How did it work?	What was achieved?
Employment of staff	Good practice resources available to practices, material available to add to job descriptions describing role around self care	Log shows all practice enquiries re help in describing self care role are dealt with satisfactorily	Responsibility for promoting and supporting self care is included in job descriptions and reviewed at annual appraisals for key personnel in all practices, community pharmacies and the PCT
Training	PCT-wide training needs analysis template includes the field of self care in relation to general practice teams and pharmacists	Training needs re promotion of self care identified on PCT-wide basis; relevant courses provided or signposted	PCT maps competence gained; case examples of staff who gain new or delegated skills are communicated and acclaimed by senior PCT staff
Strategy	Strategy for promoting and supporting self care exists, with operational plan and essential resources; strategy is a local adaptation of national policies and guidance	Senior and relevant PCT staff actively involved: i.e. senior manager in primary care, clinical governance lead, training lead; scoping exercise undertaken to map good practice; gaps identified	Evaluation of implementation of operational plan shows key indicators have been met, e.g. number of staff trained in self care, patients provided with, or signposted to resources and take-up of specific help
Standards	PCT has policy and resources to promote standards in self care: including patient safety, patient satisfaction, accessibility and accuracy of materials	Monitoring process to check that self care is being promoted, supported and adopted appropriately	PCT collation of practices' self-assessment of standards of self care show standards met 100% of the time for patient safety; 90% of the time for patient satisfaction and type of self care support resources
Patient satisfaction	Method of assessing PCT-wide patient satisfaction includes enquiry relevant to promotion and adoption of self care	Patient satisfaction assessed in respect of opportunities for convenient self care linked to general practices and community pharmacies	Changes made to supporting self care, in response to patient feedback from satisfaction survey(s)

Table 9.2: Criteria for evaluation by general practices or community pharmacies of the extent to which self care is promoted and supported across the team

Aspect of self care	What is it about?	How did it work?	What was achieved?
Employment of staff	Good practice exists e.g. material describing role with self care for new staff and updated job descriptions	Responsibility for promoting and supporting self care is reviewed at annual appraisals for key personnel in the practice or pharmacy	Good signposting recorded in pharmacy contract; appraisals reveal staff commitment to promoting and supporting patients' self care
Training	Learning needs analysis template or in-practice event exists or version that is part of PCT-wide initiative; includes field of self care in relation to the practice or pharmacy team	Training needs re promotion of self care identified throughout the practice or pharmacy; relevant course provided in-house or signposted	Practice/pharmacy maps competence gained
Skill mix	Protocol or plan for teamworking and learning in general practice/pharmacy about self care	Audits to assess if self care is being supported via teamworking protocols	Case studies or problem reviewed by practice/pharmacy shows team is working in multidisciplinary way taking on new skills in promoting and supporting self care
Standards	Practice/pharmacy has protocol to monitor standards in self care: including patient safety, patient satisfaction, accessibility and accuracy of materials	Monitoring process to check that self care is being supported and adopted appropriately	Practice/pharmacy's self-assessment of standards of self care show standards are met 100% of the time for patient safety; 90% of the time for patient satisfaction and type of self care support resources
Patient satisfaction	Method of assessing patient satisfaction includes enquiry relevant to promotion and adoption of self care e.g. OTC medicines	Patient satisfaction assessed in respect of opportunities for convenient self care linked to e.g. OTC medicines	Changes made to supporting self care, in response to patient feedback from satisfaction survey(s) e.g. OTC medicines

- was appropriate
- was safe
- was acceptable to the patient (e.g. type of treatment, frequency, fits with their religious or ethical beliefs)
- was delivered at the right time in the right way
- achieved the desired effects or outcomes
- achieved the desired outcomes with minimum effort, expense and waste.

Some examples of how you might focus on the essential components of self care support are summarised in Tables 9.1 (for a PCT) and 9.2 (for a general practice or pharmacy team). Each table has five aspects of the service relating to self care on the vertical axis, with what it is about, how it worked and what was achieved on the horizontal axis. In this example, you could generate up to 15 different aspects of the service to evaluate. Focus on several of these 15 aspects to look at the quality of self care support from various angles.

For example, if you were carrying out an evaluation of the promotion of self care you provide for people with asthma in a general practice, you might look at:

- whether patients from hard to reach groups, such as young people who receive self care advice on prevention of attacks, put advice about self care into practice and relieve worsening symptoms
- the process of communicating self care well with patients
- the extent to which a GP, nurse or pharmacist stick to the protocol to emphasise self care at successive consultations.

For each of these components you would organise a separate but linked audit.

References

1 Pawson R and Tilley N. *Realistic Evaluation*. London: Sage; 2000.
2 Chambers R and Wakley G. *Making Clinical Governance Work for You*. Oxford: Radcliffe Medical Press; 2000.

Part 2

Illustrative patient pathways to self care

You will understand the theory of this guide to promoting and supporting self care if you see it applied. The next four chapters give you examples of patient pathways in self care as applied in a typical general practice. They describe the roles that everyone in the team can play and resources you'll need – for people with sore throat, back pain, asthma, and cough and colds. There are more examples of patient pathways on the www.wipp.nhs.uk website.

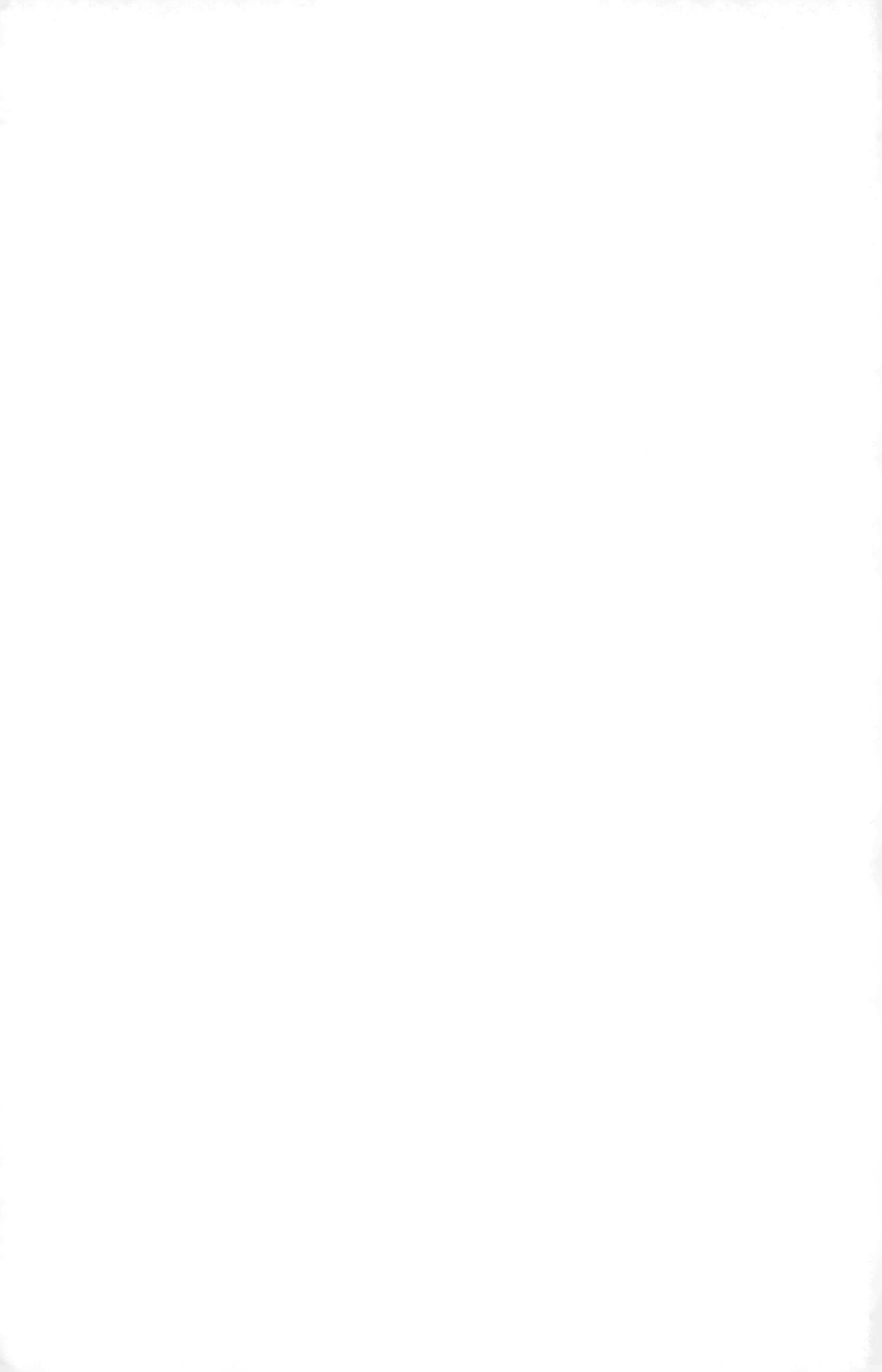

10

Illustrative patient pathway to self care: sore throat

Gill Wakley

This chapter gives you an example of a general practice team's approach to the self care of sore throat.

Section 1 Self care for sore throats

The start

We start with the patient's perspective. You could:

- work through the detailed scenario observing the sort of issues and discussion that the fictional practice team progress through here
- discuss how your team would respond to the patient story given here
- take an example case of a patient with sore throat from your own practice (anonymising the patient's identity in the team's discussion as appropriate).

If you do not know enough about the management of sore throat for completing the problem based learning, learn more about the range of self care support options and read through the clinical summary about sore throat in the second section of this chapter, before you start the problem based learning exercise.

> **Patient's story 10.1**
> 'I recently had a really bad sore throat. As I only usually have sore throats for 2–3 days, sometimes followed by a cold, I just treated this as any normal sore throat and took paracetamol as usual.
>
> A week later and I still had a sore throat, especially in the mornings, so I decided it might be time to visit the GP. I had thought of going a couple of times but know that there's not much a GP can do for a sore throat or cold and it is often advertised not to attend your GP surgery if you just have a cold.
>
> I decided to go the pharmacy first to see if they could recommend anything that would clear up my sore throat so that I didn't need to see the doctor. They sold me some medicine but it did not help my sore throat much. The next day I rang for an appointment to see the doctor. I was very impressed that I got an appointment at very short notice. I was aware, though, that by this time I had started to feel a whole lot better but as I had an appointment I thought that it was still worth going.'

> **Note**: the patient in this scenario had tried *awaiting* resolution of her symptoms, and self care for *relief* of symptoms, and to some extent was *tolerating* the symptoms.

Your project team

> Consider Tool 11 on team building

You might want a team to discuss alternative self care support options for sore throat as in this example to include:

- practice nurses
- reception staff
- practice manager
- GPs
- patient and/or carer
- pharmacist
- pharmacy assistant.

You could use a checklist as in Table 10.1 (*see* p. 130) to record who is involved and in what way.

Team discussion considering the patient story 10.1

> Consider Tools 1, 3, 4, 5, 6 or 8 for your teamwork and discussions

In this scenario, discussion between the fictional practice team members reveals:

- patients making an urgent appointment are usually seen by the GPs after the routine surgery. If a GP locum or new GP registrar is in the practice many of the urgent appointments will be with this doctor. The practice nurses are too booked up with patients with long term conditions to provide any help
- the GP's view is that many of the patients attending for urgent appointments are irritating – unless they have a serious medical complaint. The GP gives patients inadequate explanations about their condition because of the pressure of time
- the reception staff often feel squeezed between patients who are anxious about their symptoms, and the desire to reduce the burden of extra patients for the GPs. Receptionists would like more guidance to prioritise those patients who need to see a doctor urgently
- management is inconsistent. Some doctors give antibiotics for sore throats frequently, others hardly ever. None feel that they can give enough time to explain how the patient can manage next time, or how patients can decide when to consult with a sore throat. They are unsure how they would do this anyway

Illustrative patient pathway to self care: sore throat

- patients and carers continue to attend with sore throats because there is no consistent policy. They feel unsure how to take care of themselves and how long it is reasonable to wait before consulting a GP or nurse about their sore throat. They often feel that they were right to see the doctor last time because they received a prescription
- the pharmacist usually delegates advice about sore throats to the pharmacy assistants. No consistent policy has been agreed in the pharmacy. Neither have the GPs and local pharmacists agreed a policy for the treatment of sore throats and the pharmacists are unaware of which patients the GPs feel should be seen. The pharmacy assistant feels that she is expected by her employer and the customer to sell something to relieve the symptoms.

What you do next might include:

> Consider any of Tools 2, 3, 4, 5, 6, 7, 8, 9 or 10 for your action planning

- arrange a meeting between members of the primary care team and the pharmacist team to agree a common approach to supporting self care for sore throats
- nominate one of the practice nurses as the lead clinician because of her special training and skills in health promotion. (Or arrange for one of the practice nurses to receive such training before taking on the lead.) She might combine this specific task (of education about sore throats) with other prioritised health education tasks such as smoking, obesity and exercise
- examine the time that the practice nurse has available. A shortage of time will prompt an audit of tasks performed. Analysis suggests that up to 40% of the work currently performed by the practice nurse could safely be delegated to a less qualified health professional. The team decide to use an appropriately trained health care assistant. You might train suitable volunteers from the existing members of staff to the requisite standard, or employ someone already trained
- patient and carer representatives on the team help to draft and test posters and new information in the practice leaflet about the availability of advice about self care to people with sore throat, as an example.
- reception staff and pharmacy assistants will use information (see Box 10.1, p. 131) to advise patients on self care and whether they need an appointment at the surgery. Patients who are not happy with this, or who are on medication, will be referred to the nurse or doctor for telephone advice in the first instance
- the receptionists decide to give out to patients the flow chart on self care for sore throats, published by NHS Direct.[1] The practice manager will scan this into the computer so that it can easily be printed out, and check once a year that it is an up-to-date version
- the GPs and practice nurses agree to use the Prodigy patient leaflet on sore throats.[2] It can be printed out for patients who attend
- the pharmacist would prefer to use the patient information leaflet from the Scottish Intercollegiate Guidelines Network (as it does not denigrate the use of lozenges, etc

that might affect sales) and will train the pharmacist assistants on its use.[3] The pharmacy already has a supply of the leaflet on reducing antibiotic use (*Antibiotics: don't wear me out*) that customers can collect from a display[4]
- discussion about the cost of supporting self care leads to a proposal that the pharmacist and practice manager will approach the PCT. In other areas, PCTs have financed a minor ailments scheme where care is transferred from general practice to pharmacies, and patients normally exempt from prescription charges can receive OTC medicines free of charge
- the doctors and nurses agree to meet with the practice or community pharmacist to examine the evidence about the treatment of sore throats with antibiotics and to draw up an agreement so that patients receive consistent management. They will allow for patients to opt for symptomatic treatments that give them temporary reduction in the discomfort of sore throat, even if there is no or limited evidence of any particular treatment providing a 'cure'. The practice pharmacist might source the evidence, in addition to that presented in this chapter.

What extra resources might this require?

> Consider either Tool 8 or 10 for determining resource and skill needs

- Time for meetings and for training.
- Protected time for the lead practice nurse to monitor and support the introduction of the changes; time for her health promotion activities.
- Training for reception staff to use the flow chart and leaflets and direct patients to the pharmacy or practice nurse for advice.
- The practice manager will ensure that all computers are set up so that information leaflets can be printed out. A supply of ready printed leaflets will be kept in the reception area and the lead receptionist or her deputy will ensure that they are replenished.
- Additional staffing hours may be needed initially – achieved by modifying the workload of existing staff, extending the hours of existing staff or employing additional staff. An additional health care assistant may be the most cost effective approach.
- Schemes for transfer of management of minor ailments funded by PCTs have allocated funding for a pharmacy facilitator for setting up the scheme. The PCT needs to fund the cost of the medicine supplied plus a consultation fee for the pharmacist.
- The pharmacy may need extra time, but many of the consultations in minor ailments schemes are basically transfers from dispensing of a prescription that the patient would have received from a doctor. There should be an area to preserve the confidentiality of consultations between the pharmacist and patients, and assistance with the paperwork created by the minor ailments scheme.
- Supplies of leaflets and posters about the minor ailments scheme.

The outcomes might include:

> Either of Tools 9 or 12 will help to monitor progress

- better and more confident self care of sore throats by patients and carers (P, A, R, T) (**P**revent the condition, **A**wait resolution, use self care for **R**elief of symptoms, learn to **T**olerate symptoms) *see* Box 10.1, p. 131
- fewer requests for GP appointments from patients with sore throats (A, R, T)
- a decrease in the number of patients prescribed antibiotics (A, R, T)
- no failures to identify those few patients requiring medical input (R).

How would you demonstrate that you have achieved your outcomes?

> Consider Tools 9 and 12 for reviewing outcomes

- Record GP appointments for sore throats before and at intervals after the project, to demonstrate changes in demand.
- Record the lead practice nurse's appointments for giving self care advice on sore throats before and at intervals after the project, to demonstrate changes in demand.
- Record numbers of patients seen at the pharmacy for advice before and at intervals after the project, to demonstrate changes in demand.
- Record the number and type of patients referred from the pharmacist, pharmacy assistants, practice nurse(s) and receptionists for medical care of sore throat.
- Conduct a significant event examination of any complaint, missed diagnosis or adverse outcome subsequent to the change to self care support or pharmacy advice.

Table 10.1: Role and responsibilities checklist

For each task tick the box for each team member who has a role or responsibility – then note your role and responsibilities for the task.

Completed by ______________________________

Task	*Doctor*	*Practice nurse*	*Patient or carer*	*Reception team*	*Practice manager*	*Practice based or community pharmacist*	*Pharmacy assistant*	*PCT*	*What are the roles and responsibilities?*
	Project team member								
Promoting the concept of self care, issuing leaflets, redirecting patients to pharmacy advice	✓	✓		✓	✓	✓	✓	✓	Every person seen complaining of a sore throat can be supplied with self care information
Recording attendances	✓	✓		✓		✓	✓		To ensure self care advice given to patients consulting with sore throat is recorded so that the advice is reinforced at any similar consultation in the future
Significant event audit	✓	✓	(✓)	✓	✓	✓	✓		Any serious missed diagnosis or adverse outcome relating to the management of sore throat is examined
Agree protocol for supporting self care of sore throat	✓	✓			✓	✓		✓	Discussions with PCT re justifying and setting up of minor ailments scheme; practice protocol agreed with local pharmacist meanwhile
Task 5 – you add									

Section 2 Self care for sore throats

How big is the problem?

Sore throat is a common reason for people to seek medical attention. A GP with 2000 patients will see around 120 people with acute throat infections every year.[5] Most people with sore throat do not attend their GP.[6] Young people and children are the most frequent attenders, especially in winter.

Symptoms

Pain in the throat and on swallowing is the most common complaint. Fever, headache, a white or grey covering over the back of the throat, swollen glands below the jaw and at the sides of the neck, feeling or being sick, and abdominal pain may be present. Cough, a runny nose or a hoarse voice often occur together with a sensation of a sore throat, and suggest a viral cause. Throat infections usually improve over three to seven days.[7]

Self care advice and guidance: take PART

Think of the range of advice and guidance about self care you might give to patients who consult you with a sore throat. *See* Box 10.1.

Box 10.1: Range of self care advice and guidance for sore throat you can give to patients or carers

P *Prevention*: it is difficult to avoid catching infections from other people. Washing your hands more frequently, especially after blowing or touching your nose, can reduce the spread of germs by hand contact. Try to avoid standing too close to someone with an obvious cold or sore throat. Avoid sharing drinking or eating utensils with others.

A *Await* resolution of the symptoms: a sore throat usually cures itself in three to seven days, but may take longer if associated with a cold or cough. Ask your pharmacist or call NHS Direct if you are not sure how to take care of it.

R Use self care for *relief* of symptoms: drink fluids (not alcohol) in small amounts frequently. Take pain relief, if needed, such as paracetamol in the recommended dose on the container – that could be the maximum dose on days when the pain is most severe. Taking painkillers regularly helps to keep the pain under control. Avoid foods that cause discomfort when swallowed; ice cream and soft foods often help. Gargling with salt water or sucking lozenges eases throat soreness. Avoid smoking and smoky atmospheres.

T Learn to *tolerate* symptoms that do not resolve or cannot be reasonably alleviated. Increasing rest periods helps your body to get on with healing itself.

> **When they should seek further advice**
>
> Tell them:
>
> If you have any of the following speak to NHS Direct (0845 4647) or a doctor or nurse at your general practice surgery:
>
> - you have a sore throat lasting more than two weeks, difficulty in swallowing or a hoarse voice
> - you feel generally unwell with tender lumps in your armpits and groin as well as in your neck
> - you have a rash and a fever
> - you have any difficulty breathing or swallowing your own saliva.

Alarm symptoms or signs (red flags)

Quinsy

Symptoms include a worsening sore throat, usually on one side, with fever, difficulty opening the mouth, difficulty swallowing, drooling rather than swallowing their own saliva and sometimes swelling of the face and neck. It requires urgent medical assessment and, if confirmed, rapid referral to hospital for surgical drainage.

Epiglottitis

The first symptoms are a high temperature and rapid onset of a very sore throat. Severe difficulty in swallowing follows, with drooling, spitting, fast and very noisy breathing. A child will sit straight upright in order to help them breathe more easily, or may sit with their chin forward. In infants there may be problems with sucking when breast or bottle feeding.

As the epiglottis swells and blocks the airways, a child may find it hard to breathe, and their skin may turn grey or blue. They may be restless and panicky, and have fever or shivering attacks. They may be unable to speak or have a very muffled voice, make grunting type noises and sit leaning forward, trying to keep their airways open. Never lie the child down or try to look in their throat, as this can trigger a spasm that closes their throat completely, and can cause death within a few minutes. In adults, symptoms are similar, but they start more gradually and recovery is usually slower. The main symptom is usually severe pain that is worse on swallowing.

This condition is an emergency, and you should phone 999 for an emergency ambulance, or get the affected person to the nearest A&E department.

Agranulocytosis

The commonest causes are drug reactions or infections in already immuno-compromised patients. Patients taking drugs commonly associated with this adverse reaction should have received warnings to report sore throats promptly, and need medical evaluation.

Other diagnoses

Glandular fever

Sore throat with fever, feeling unwell generally, and swollen glands in the neck, armpit and groin may suggest glandular fever, otherwise known as infectious mononucleosis or Epstein–Barr virus (EBV). Abdominal pain and a rash may also occur and the spleen may be enlarged. A blood test can confirm the diagnosis and symptomatic treatment advised.

Scarlet fever

The main symptoms include sore throat with fever, headache, vomiting and swollen neck glands. The tongue has a thick white coating that peels to leave a red 'strawberry' appearance. The rash usually appears on the second day and looks like sunburn. You can feel little bumps all over it and it may be itchy. It appears on the neck, and spreads to the rest of the body. The skin affected may peel off, especially around the fingers and toes. The causative agent is the toxin produced by the group A beta-haemolytic streptococcus (GABHS).

Persistent sore throat

Consider other diagnoses such as perennial or seasonal rhinitis with postnasal catarrh, and, rarely, blood abnormalities like leukaemia.

Late complications

Other complications of acute sore throat caused by GABHS are sinusitis or otitis media.
Non-suppurative complications include acute nephritis and rheumatic fever, both now very rare in developed countries.

Identifying GABHS

Throat swab cultures can take 24–48 hours to be reported, limiting their usefulness for a decision during the consultation. The high rate of asymptomatic carriers in the population of around 40% means that many people with a positive throat culture will not have a sore throat caused by GABHS.[5] Rapid antigen testing gives a quick result in the consultation, but still only tells you if GABHS is present, not if it is the cause. Neither is much help with deciding on whether to treat with antibiotics!

A symptom and sign score such as the Centor score may help to decide whether GABHS is present using the criteria:[8,9]

- tonsillar exudates
- tender anterior cervical lymph nodes
- fever
- absence of cough.

A score of 0, 1 or 2 of the criteria shows low likelihood of GABHS infection; a score of 3 or 4 of the criteria increases the likelihood of GABHS infection.

Using antibiotics

A study in children using two of the Centor criteria as the cut off point for treating with antibiotics showed that antibiotics did not help the symptoms but did reduce the complications of imminent quinsy, impetigo and scarlet fever.[10] However, the authors did not advise immediate prescription of antibiotics even for this group of children who were more unwell. Delayed antibiotic use in children whose illness worsened was sufficient. A commentary on this and other studies concluded that seven children with two of the four Centor criteria would have to be treated to prevent one case of worsening of illness.[11] The other six would suffer the disadvantages of side-effects, reduced local and systemic immunity and the cycle of recurrence.

A systematic review by the Cochrane Collaboration suggested that antibiotics might shorten the length of time symptoms persisted, but only by eight hours overall.[12] Around 90% of patients were symptom free after seven days, whether or not they received antibiotics. There was no evidence that treatment with antibiotics resulted in an earlier return to school or work. The review also reported that, although antibiotic treatment reduced the incidence of otitis media and sinusitits, this did not translate into significant clinical benefits. To prevent one episode of otitis media, about 30 children and 145 adults with sore throat would need to be treated with antibiotics.

Other studies have reported the lack of success in preventing both rheumatic fever and acute glomerulonephritits when sore throats were treated with antibiotics. Most clinical trials have used 10 days of penicillin or erythromycin to eradicate GABHS. It is not clear if shorter courses are any less effective in relieving symptoms or preventing complications.[5] Other antibiotics such as amoxicillin should be avoided because of the risk of precipitating a rash if the patient has glandular fever.

The *MeRec Bulletin* and the SIGN guidelines both conclude that GPs should avoid prescribing antibiotics for most sore throats.[5,6] In very ill patients, or those with a history of previous complication, penicillin or erythromycin may be used. A delayed prescription, to be used if symptoms worsen after a few days, may be a useful compromise for patients unconvinced by an explanation of the evidence. There are two models for a 'delayed' prescription: one where the patient comes back to the practice if the condition persists,[13] and the other where a post-dated prescription is given.[14] In any audit you undertake of your prescribing for sore throats, you should develop a system to account for delayed antibiotic prescriptions not presented to the pharmacy because the person's sore throat symptoms have resolved. If the prescription is left at the practice to collect, you should delete it as having been issued, on your computer system. If you opt for the post-dated delayed prescription model, see if you can allocate a specific code for delayed prescriptions via your practice computer system.

Apart from being mainly unnecessary or ineffective for sore throat, prescribing antibiotics can trigger a learnt behaviour resulting in future unnecessary consultations.

Find a way to gain everyone's agreement on your policy for prescribing antibiotics in general, and in this instance for sore throat – and review the extent to which all prescribers are adhering to your practice policy. Advertise that message to patients so they know when they should consult a doctor or nurse with their sore throat or when they might benefit from an antibiotic. This might be a central part of establishing a local minor ailments scheme in pharmacies and general practices (*see* Chapter 6).

References

1. www.nhsdirect.nhs.uk/SelfHelpGuide
2. www.prodigy.nhs.uk
3. www.sign.ac.uk/guidelines/fulltext/34/annex2.html
4. Department of Health. *Antibiotics: don't wear me out*. London: Department of Health; 2005. www.dh.gov.uk/assetRoot/04/05/71/75/04057175.pdf
5. National Prescribing Centre. Managing sore throats. *MeReC Bulletin*. 1999; **10 (11)**.
6. SIGN. *Management of Sore Throat and Indications for Tonsillectomy: a national clinical guideline*. Report No. 34. Edinburgh: Scottish Intercollegiate Guidelines Network; 1999. www.sign.ac.uk
7. Prodigy guidance: www.prodigy.nhs.uk/pk.uk/sore_throat_acute/
8. McIsaac W, White D, Tannenbaum D and Low DE. A clinical score to reduce unnecessary antibiotic use in patients with sore throat. *Canadian Medical Association Journal*. 1998; **158**: 75–83.
9. McIsaac W, Goel V, To T and Low DE. The validity of a sore throat score in family practice. *Canadian Medical Association Journal*. 2000; **163**: 811–15.
10. Zwart S, Poever MM, de Melker RA *et al*. Penicillin for acute sore throat in children: randomised, double blind trail. *British Medical Journal*. 2003; **327**: 1324–7.
11. Little P. More valid criteria may be needed. *British Medical Journal*. 2003; **327**: 1327–8.
12. Del Mar CB and Glasziou PP. Antibiotics for sore throat (Cochrane Review). The Cochrane Library, Issue 3. Oxford: Update Software; 1999.
13. Little P, Williamson I, Warner G *et al*. Open randomised trial of prescribing strategies in managing sore throat. *British Medical Journal*. 1997; **314**: 722–7.
14. Edwards M, Dennison J and Sedgwick P. Patients' responses to delayed antibiotic prescription for acute upper respiratory tract infections. *British Journal of General Practice*. 2003; **53**: 845–50.

11

Illustrative patient pathway to self care: back pain
Gill Wakley

This chapter gives you an example of a practice team's approach to the self care of back pain.

Section 1 Self care for back pain

The start

We start with a patient's perspective. You could:

- work through the detailed scenario observing the sort of issues and discussion that the fictional practice team progress through here
- discuss how your team would respond to the patient story given here
- take an example case of a patient with back pain from your own practice (anonymising the patient's identity in the team's discussion as appropriate).

If you feel that you do not know enough about the management of back pain to complete the problem based learning, then learn more about the range of self care support options and clinical summary about back pain in the second section of this chapter before you start the problem based learning exercise.

> **Patient's story 11.1**
> After four days of severe back pain, Barbara thought she should make an appointment to see the doctor. Unfortunately, Barbara was uneasy as the doctor hardly examined her. The examination consisted of a light touch to her side asking if it hurt and then before Barbara could explain any further he had turned away and started to prescribe strong painkillers.
>
> Around two months later Barbara was still having back pain and decided that she would see a different doctor. This time blood tests were done and Barbara felt as though she had been looked after and listened to. Nothing more was discussed around Barbara's back pain this time as the blood test showed a different problem that needed to be treated as a matter of urgency.
>
> Barbara carried on taking the strong painkillers for her back pain prescribed by the first doctor and also rubbed in Ibuleve which she bought herself. She bought an exercise machine to help her with exercising but this did not help.
>
> Barbara will try visiting the doctor again, but doesn't feel that she has had much help with taking care of her back pain so far.

Illustrative patient pathway to self care: back pain 137

> **Note**: the patient in this scenario had tried *awaiting* resolution of her symptoms, and self care with Ibuleve for *relief* of symptoms, then *prevention* to some extent with the exerciser, and finally *tolerating* the back pain in some measure, though unhappily.

Your project team

> Consider Tool 11 on team building

You might want a team to discuss alternative self care support options for back pain as in this example, to include:

- reception staff
- practice manager
- GPs
- practice nurses
- health visitor
- midwife
- district nurses
- patient and/or carer
- physiotherapist
- practice secretary
- community pharmacist
- practice-based pharmacist.

You could use a checklist as in Table 11.1 (*see* p. 141) to record who is involved and in what way.

Team discussion considering the patient story 11.1

> Consider Tools 1, 3, 4, 5, 6, 8 or 10 for your teamwork and discussions

In this scenario, discussion between the fictional practice team members reveals:

- GPs view many of the patients attending for back pain as a nuisance. They think patients should take care of their acute back pain themselves and tend to feel that many people with chronic back pain are trying to avoid activity or using it for secondary gain. But they are fearful of encouraging patients with back pain to do self care and missing something serious
- management is inconsistent. Some doctors give codeine-based analgesics routinely, others think a combination of paracetamol and a non-steroidal anti-inflammatory drug (NSAID) better. None feel that they can give enough time to explain how the patient can take care of the pain themselves, or how patients can

decide when to consult with back pain. They are unsure how they would do this anyway. They would like to give patients a booklet but think copies of *The Back Book* are too expensive to give away[1]
- the practice has some books, tapes and videos to loan to patients. Many of these have disappeared and there is no formal scheme for recording who has what. No patient information materials on back care are in stock
- receptionists feel that patients with back pain are anxious and in pain and need to see the doctor. Receptionists would like to prioritise those patients who need to see a doctor
- patients continue to attend with back pain because there is no consistent policy. They feel unsure how to take care of themselves and that they were right to see the doctor because they received a prescription or investigations
- practice nurses always refer patients with back pain to the GP as they do not feel competent to advise them
- the midwife, district nurses and health visitor have had specific training and education about how to prevent and advise on self care for mechanical lower back pain, and feel that the rest of the team is simply not up to speed
- the physiotherapist reports that too many people with back pain, who really just need information, are referred inappropriately for physiotherapy. The long waiting list means that, by the time they are seen, most of them have either recovered, or are fixed in a pattern of avoidance of any movement that hurts
- the community pharmacist reports that people often ask for 'something stronger' than simple painkillers, and options available OTC are limited because doses of codeine and dihydrocodeine are lower than in prescription medicines. The practice pharmacist wants to discuss the GPs' prescribing of topical NSAIDs, for which she says there is insufficient evidence in most cases.

What you do next might include:

> Consider any of Tools 2, 3, 4, 5, 6, 7, 8, 9 or 10 for your action planning

- arrange a meeting between all members of the team to agree a common approach to promoting prevention and supporting self care for acute back pain
- the health visitor agrees to lead the project team as she feels competent to advise on prevention and self care of back pain from her special training and education, and can act as a resource for other team members. Fortunately, she is based in the practice and is readily available. One of the district nurses with similar training agrees to act as her deputy
- the practice manager agrees to consider whether a health care assistant might help the health visitor to free up some time
- the practice manager will act as the convenor of meetings and training and ensure that any decisions and training are rolled out to all staff
- the practice secretary will formalise the loaning of information to patients. Useful books,[2,3] videos/DVDs will be purchased and the receptionists trained in how to

record who has what and when loan items are taken and returned. The secretary will review the record cards each month and write to those people who have overdue items
- the practice manager liaises with the local library to find out if there is a facility for dealing with enquiries about health, or any formal scheme with which the practice can link
- the patient representative helps to draft and test posters and new information in the practice leaflet about the availability of advice about prevention and self care
- the receptionists decide to use the flow chart published by NHS Direct.[4] The practice manager will scan this into the computer so that it can easily be accessed or printed out
- the practice will apply to the PCT for extra funding for supplies of *The Back Book* so that all patients with acute back pain can collect a copy.[1] Patients who are not happy with this will be referred to the doctor, health visitor or district nurse for telephone advice in the first instance
- the doctors and physiotherapist agree to meet to examine the literature about the management of back pain and to put a guideline on the practice computer screen so that patients receive consistent care.[5] They become aware of patients' dissatisfaction in general with the amount and quality of information and advice they receive, particularly regarding diagnosis and treatment.[6] While meeting they review websites they can recommend to patients as having sound advice about back care – including back exercises and equipment; the practice secretary prepares a printout for patients signposting these recommended websites
- the physiotherapist agrees to run back care prevention and self care classes for all staff on two different days to ensure that all can attend.

What extra resources might this require?

> Consider either Tool 8, 10 or 17 for determining resource and skill needs

- Time for meetings and for training.
- Protected time for the practice manager to arrange meetings and training, monitor and support the introduction of changes.
- Training for the reception staff in the use of the flow chart and booklet.
- Training for reception staff on the loan scheme.
- Time for the practice secretary to chase up overdue items from the loan scheme and to audit referrals.
- Time (and possibly training) for staff to implement, monitor and audit the project.
- Additional staffing hours may be needed initially – through modifying the workload of existing staff, extending the hours of existing staff or employing additional staff. An additional health care assistant may be the most cost effective approach.
- The back pain prevention and self care classes will be in paid protected time for the staff.

The outcomes might include:

> Either of Tools 9 or 12 will help to monitor progress

- better and more confident self care of back pain by patients and carers (A, R, T) (**P**revent the condition, **A**wait resolution, use self care for **R**elief of symptoms, learn to **T**olerate symptoms) *see* Box 11.1, p. 142)
- fewer episodes of back pain in those who have received information about prevention (P)
- fewer requests for GP appointments from patients with back pain (P, A, R, T)
- improvement in the care of acute, sub-acute and chronic back pain by GPs (A, R, T)
- fewer inappropriate referrals to the physiotherapy service resulting in a more targeted service (A, R, T)
- fewer referrals to secondary care orthopaedic or pain services because of more confident and expert management by GPs and self care by patients (A, R, T)
- no failures to identify and refer those few patients requiring medical input for acute back pain (A, R)

How would you demonstrate that you have achieved your outcomes?

> Consider Tools 9 or 12 for reviewing outcomes

- Feedback (informal and formal) from patients and carers about their self care of back pain.
- Practice manager records absences for back pain among staff before and after the back care classes, and examines any episodes sustained at work for avoidable factors.
- Comparison of the rates of re-attendance with further episodes of back pain among those patients who attended with a first attack before and after the introduction of the information about prevention, management and self care.
- Comparison of consultation rates for back pain before and after the project.
- Self-rating and peer discussion of the care of acute, sub-acute and chronic back pain by GPs.
- Comparison of referrals rated as inappropriate by the physiotherapy service before and after the project.
- Comparison of the number and types of referrals to secondary care orthopaedic or pain services before and after the project.
- Significant event audit of any failures to identify and refer those few patients requiring medical input for acute back pain.

Illustrative patient pathway to self care: back pain

Table 11.1: Role and responsibilities checklist

For each task tick the box for each team member who has a role or responsibility – then note your role and responsibilities for the task.

Completed by _____

Task	Health visitor and district nurse	Practice manager	Patient or carer	Reception team	GPs	Physiotherapist	Practice secretary	Practice based or community pharmacist	What are the roles and responsibilities?
Provision of information	✓	✓		✓	✓	✓	✓	✓	Every person with acute back pain can be supplied with self care information
Care of back pain		✓			✓	✓			Ensure consistent and up-to-date care of acute and chronic back pain
Significant event audit	✓	✓	(✓)	✓	✓	✓	✓		Any complaint, missed diagnosis or adverse outcome is examined in relation to patients consulting with back pain
Audit of referrals to physiotherapy, orthopaedic and pain services		✓			✓	✓	✓		Examination of the appropriateness of the referral of patients with back pain, the extent to which self care had been advocated and supported, discussion of the comparison of before and after referrals, plan and implementation of action for any change
Task 5 – you add									

Section 2 Self care for back pain

How big is the problem?

Around 4% of consultations with GPs are for low back pain. More than seven out of ten people in developed countries will have back pain at some time in their lives and between 15% and 45% of adults suffer low back pain each year.[5] Around 4.9 million working days are lost due to back pain every year, costing British industry billions of pounds.[7] Around 70% of people who are on sickness absence due to back pain will return to work within one week, and 90% return within two months. The longer the period of sickness absence with back pain, the less likely it is that someone will return to work.

Symptoms

Pain and muscle tightness or stiffness in the back between the lower ribs and the top of the legs is the commonest complaint. Pain going down the leg (sciatica) may be present. Back pain is classified into:

- *acute*: lasting under six weeks
- *sub-acute*: lasting between 6 and 12 weeks
- *chronic*: lasting more than 12 weeks.

Symptoms, pathology and X-ray appearances are poorly correlated and most people have non-specific mechanical pain that cannot be accurately categorised. About 4% of people with low back pain have compression fractures and around 1% have tumours. A prolapsed intervertebral disc is only present in 1–3%. Ankylosing spondylitis and infections are rare.[5]

Risk factors

Back pain is more likely in those people who do heavy physical work, frequent bending, twisting and lifting, suffer whole body vibration, or remain in one position for a long time. Psychosocial factors (often known as 'yellow flags') include anxiety, depression and mental stress at work. Most people developing low back pain are adults aged 20–55 years and are otherwise well.[7]

Self care advice and guidance: take PART

Think of the range of advice and guidance about self care you might give to patients who consult you with back pain (*see* Box 11.1).

> **Box 11.1:** Range of self care advice and guidance for back pain to give to patients or their carers
>
> **P** Programmes for the general public for the *prevention* of back pain are mainly run by public health, governmental organisations, voluntary agencies and employers. PCTs, general practice teams, pharmacies, and other health care departments may want to run their own prevention programmes.

Workplace initiatives can help to prevent back pain, the commonest form of ill health at work.[7] Education projects in schools can help children to be more aware of their posture, how they use their backs and what causes back pain.[8] Midwives,[9] district nurses and health visitors can educate individuals or groups. GPs, physiotherapists and other physical therapists who see people who have already had an episode of back pain, can help people to avoid recurrences.[10,11] Avoiding manual lifting by using machines and aids, learning to lift properly and how to stand and sit with proper support, as well as flexibility and strengthening exercises should be included in the programmes.

A *Await* resolution: most people with acute back pain have sufficient improvements in pain and disability to return to work within one month. Further improvements occur up to three months, after which pain and disability remain almost constant. Low levels of pain and disability may persist from three to at least 12 months. Most people will have at least one recurrence within 12 months.[12] A safety net of advice on warning signs of more serious conditions is needed.[13] You could use the algorithm on self care for backache in adults produced by NHS Direct.[4]

R Advice on self care for *relief* of symptoms (*see* Box 11.2).

T Many of the activities suggested above are also applicable to *tolerating* symptoms from long term back pain: *Clinical Evidence* provides evidence for various strategies to care for chronic back pain.[5]

Box 11.2: Advice on relief of symptoms by self care of back pain to give to patients or their carers

- Take it easy for the first couple of days, move about gently, avoid bending forward, avoid strain and don't sit in a chair for any length of time. Take painkillers like paracetamol or ibuprofen according to the manufacturer's instructions. A heat or ice pack applied to your lower back for around 30 minutes may help. Wrap ice packs in a towel.
- Keep active and move around even if it hurts. Small amounts of exercise very frequently are best. Specific exercises done within the limits of the pain can be helpful. A book or website on back care or advice from a physiotherapist, osteopath or chiropractor can guide you in what exercises would be beneficial.
- If the pain persists, physical treatment from a physiotherapist, osteopath or chiropractor can help you to get moving. Pilates, massage or acupuncture may help.
- Read up on relief of back pain in these helpful books:
  - Burton K. *The Back Book*. London: The Stationery Office; 2002.
  - Chambers R. *Beat Back Pain* (52 brilliant ideas series). Oxford: The Infinite Ideas Company Ltd; 2005.
  - McKenzie R. *Treat Your Own Back*. Lower Hutt, New Zealand: Spinal Publications Ltd; 1997. www.backcare.org.uk/

Alarm symptoms or signs (red flags)

- Age outside the usual range should prompt a medical review for causes other than simple mechanical pain. Mechanical back pain in children is more common than previously thought; around 13% of teenagers experience recurrent mechanical low back pain.[14]
- Associated pain in the abdomen with a pulsating sensation; or pain in the chest and upper back made worse by a severe cough or wheeze (may be a dissecting aneurysm – especially in someone over 60 years old).
- Presence of fever or rigors (shivering attacks), being generally unwell, loss of weight or severe unrelenting pain, including at night, suggests infection or cancer.
- Pain that worsens with walking, that goes into both legs, with or without leg weakness, and is associated with relief by bending forward, may be due to spinal stenosis and should be referred urgently to secondary care.
- Radiation of pain into both legs may be due to a central disc herniation, cancer or an inflammatory condition, and requires further investigation.
- Numbness in the genital area and around the back passage, incontinence or difficulty with bladder or bowel emptying, or muscle weakness may be due to spinal cord compression, and requires immediate referral.
- A history of recent injury, HIV infection or other immunosuppression or a past history of cancer requires further investigation.
- Persistent pain and stiffness in a person under 40 years old suggests spondylitis.

Other diagnoses

If other symptoms accompany the back pain, for example, burning when passing urine, a pain that moves from one side of the back to the groin, upper back pain with a cough and fever, assessment by a health practitioner is required. A long list of differential diagnoses for back pain accompanied by other symptoms appears in the Prodigy guidelines.[14]

Investigations

Taking an X-ray of the lumbar spine is not useful in mechanical low back pain. X-rays expose the patient to harmful radiation and increase the workload and costs for the NHS with no improvement in clinical outcomes. Magnetic resonance imaging is the best procedure if symptoms and signs suggest nerve root compression or a tumour. Blood tests may be indicated if an inflammatory or neoplastic condition is suspected.

Treatments

- Advice to remain active has been shown to be the most effective treatment. Bed rest is worse than no treatment.[5]
- Paracetamol is the first choice for pain relief because the risk of adverse effects is low, it is inexpensive and effective for mild pain. Codeine-containing pain relief is the next step up the pain control ladder.[5]

- NSAIDs have been shown to increase overall improvement after one week and reduce the need for additional analgesia.[5]
- Cognitive behavioural therapy reduces acute low back pain and disability by addressing psychosocial factors.[5]
- Muscle relaxants can be helpful for short term use, but there are dangers of dependence, dizziness and drowsiness, especially with benzodiazepines.[5]
- Chronic back pain is usually treated with analgesics including opioids, antidepressants (most trials have used amitriptyline) and NSAIDs. Non-drug treatments such as spinal manipulation, back schools, exercise or physical conditioning treatment are likely to help. A summary of the evidence for other treatments appears in *Clinical Evidence*.[13]

References

1 Burton K. *The Back Book*. London: The Stationery Office; 2002.

2 Chambers R. *Beat Back Pain* (52 brilliant ideas series). Oxford: The Infinite Ideas Company Ltd; 2005.

3 McKenzie R. *Treat Your Own Back*. New Zealand: Spinal Publications Ltd; 1997.

4 www.nhsdirect.nhs.uk

5 Tovey D (ed). *Clinical Evidence Concise (13)*. London: BMJ Publishing Group; 2005. www.clinicalevidence.com/ceweb/conditions/msd/1102/1102.jsp

6 McIntosh A and Shaw C. Barriers to patient information provision in primary care: patients' and general practitioners' experiences and expectations of information for low back pain. *Health Expectations*. 2003; **6:** 19–29.

7 www.hse.gov.uk/msd/backpain

8 Airedale Physiotherapy Clinic. *The Airedale Backcare for Children programme*. In: Chartered Society of Physiotherapists. *Making Physiotherapy Count*. London: Chartered Society of Physiotherapists; 2004. www.csp.org.uk/sepp

9 www.pregnancy.com.au/back_pain_in_pregnancy.htm

10 www.positivehealth.com/permit/Articles/Back%20Pain/ablett24.htm

11 www.nhsdirect.nhs.uk/en.aspx?ArticleID=234

12 Pengel LHM, Herbert RD, Maher CG and Refshauge KM. Acute low back pain: systematic review of its prognosis. *British Medical Journal*. 2003; **327:** 323–5.

13 www.clinicalevidence.com/ceweb/conditions/msd/1116/1116.jsp?searchTerm=chronic+back+pain

14 www.prodigy.nhs.uk/pk.uk/back_pain_lower

12

Illustrative patient pathway to self care: asthma
Gill Wakley

This chapter gives you an example of a practice team's approach to the self care of asthma.

Section 1 Self care for asthma

The start

We start from a patient's perspective. You could:

- work through the detailed scenario observing the sort of issues and discussion that the fictional practice team progress through here
- discuss how your team would respond to the patient story given here
- take an example case of a patient with asthma from your own practice (anonymising the patient's identity in the team's discussion as appropriate).

If you feel that you do not know enough about the management of asthma to complete the problem based learning, learn more about the range of self care support options and read through the clinical summary about asthma in the second section of this chapter before you start the problem based learning exercise.

Patient's story 12.1

'I have recently moved house and registered with another health practice. This one seems more interested in supporting people like me to look after themselves better.

Before I met with the asthma nurse for the first time, I had only been to one asthma clinic at my last practice. This was probably partly my fault as I was reluctant to go there unless I was ill and I did not think that my asthma was severe enough to warrant getting time off work just for a check up. The practice I am with now sends me an invitation to make an appointment to review my asthma. The letter acts as a reminder. It makes me feel that I am not wasting their time by going when I'm not ill.

It wasn't until my first appointment with the new practice that I realised what a mess my asthma was in. I had no control over it and must have got used to living with it that way. The nurse got me to do a peak flow reading and asked a variety of questions which led to the conclusion that I was not using my inhalers properly. The nurse prescribed a spacer for me, explained how to use it

Illustrative patient pathway to self care: asthma

and which inhaler to use with it, and asked me to try this for about a month and a half. While I was there, the nurse made an appointment for me to go back so she could monitor my progress.

After a few visits to see the nurse, I was able to report that my asthma had improved a lot and I was much more in control of it. This has made such a difference to my quality of life. The nurse filled in a plan for how I could take care of my asthma in future, which I took home with me. I can look at my self care plan on the card when I'm not sure what to do.'

Note: the patient in this scenario had needlessly *awaited* resolution of and *tolerated* the symptoms, and after coaching can do self care for their asthma to *relieve* the symptoms and *prevent* it worsening.

Your project team

Consider Tool 11 on team building

You might want a team to discuss alternative self care support options for asthma as in this example, to include:

- reception staff
- practice manager
- GPs
- practice nurses
- health care assistants
- practice-based pharmacist
- district nurse
- patient representative
- physiotherapist
- practice secretary.

You could use a checklist as in Table 12.1 (*see* p. 151), to record who is involved and in what way.

Team discussion considering the patient story 12.1

Consider Tools 1, 3, 4, 5, 6, 8 or 10 for your teamwork and discussions

In this scenario, discussion between the fictional practice team members reveals:
- the pharmacist is keen to be involved in supporting self care of asthma. She has been concerned about the high level of symptoms she hears about and the number

of people who appear to be using reliever inhalers without preventer inhalers. She would like to be involved in asthma reviews, but is worried about the time involved
- the doctors and nurses manage asthma following the British Thoracic Society and SIGN guidelines (or in the USA those from the National Heart Lung and Blood Institute's Practical Guide for the Diagnosis and Management of Asthma) but concordance with treatment is poor[1-3]
- practice nurses who have been trained in asthma management are still catching up with making sure all the people using inhalers have a diagnosis of asthma or chronic obstructive pulmonary disease (COPD). They have insufficient time to educate people about asthma or how to take care of it themselves
- health care assistants would like to be involved in asthma management but lack training. The nurses feel that they do not have time to do any training
- receptionists involved in repeat prescriptions complain that doctors give further prescriptions to patients on repeat medication for inhalers even when they have ignored requests to come for review
- receptionists feel anxious about how they should deal with patients who need help with acute asthma
- the district nurse complains that patients who are housebound are not receiving the same reviews as those able to attend the surgery
- the patient representative feels patients are made to feel that they must ask the experts how to take care of their asthma. He feels that a small panel of patients who have experience of undertaking self care for their asthma could help educate others
- the physiotherapist sends a message to say that she is unable to see people with asthma breathing dysfunction as she has insufficient appointment time
- the practice manager is concerned about the wasted time in asthma clinics when people do not attend. The practice secretary feels that the practice nurses should be responsible for recalling patients to the asthma clinic and it wastes secretarial time sending out appointments that are not kept.

What you do next might include:

> Consider any of Tools 2, 3, 4, 5, 6, 7, 8, 9 or 10 for your action planning

- arrange a meeting for the members of the project team to look at ways that patients can be educated about prevention of attacks following their self care plans
- the practice manager and practice nurses agree to consider how the health care assistants can extend their role to relieve the practice nurses of some of the recording work in the asthma clinic and of the time-consuming activity of teaching the use of inhalers
- the practice manager will ask if the physiotherapist can come to the practice to teach the practice team about hyperventilation and how to control breathing
- two receptionists will be trained to send patients a computer-generated letter explaining why review is necessary and inviting them to make an appointment instead of sending them a fixed appointment. A computer audit search will be done

each month to identify the patients after the practice secretary has set this up from her present recall system
- one of the GPs will form a small group of patient educators. He has recently been to a workshop about using patients as educators in registrar training and is enthusiastic to extend the principle. The aim will be to run regular meetings for people with asthma at a suitable venue, with minimal input from professionals
- the practice manager will arrange a workshop for the receptionists to go through various clinical scenarios and learn the difference between the zones of control of asthma in patients' self care plans
- district nurses agree to have training from the asthma-trained practice nurses
- the district nurses and the practice will negotiate with the district nurse manager for time to review housebound patients that they already visit, as the numbers are small
- receptionists will compile a list of patients who are housebound but requiring review. The practice manager will approach a voluntary service that provides hospital and day care transport to see if these few people could be brought to the practice for review
- the practice nurse will trial a buddying scheme, where newly diagnosed patients with asthma are paired with someone of similar age and background whose asthma was diagnosed a while ago and is under good control
- the practice-based pharmacist and practice manager will approach the PCT to propose that patients with asthma are a target group for MURs by community pharmacists, as these reviews are paid for from the national pharmacy budget. The reviews will last about 20–25 minutes and focus on how patients are using medicines and their understanding of their treatment (e.g. asthma). These will be annual reviews with additional reviews as required.

What extra resources might this require?

> Consider either Tool 8, 10 or 17 for determining resource and skill needs

- Time for meetings and for training.
- Protected time for the practice manager to arrange meetings and training, monitor and support the introduction of the changes.
- Physiotherapist time to come to the practice to run an education session.
- Protected time for the receptionists to operate the recall system.
- Time for the GP to set up and support the patient educators and asthma group.
- Longer appointments in the asthma clinic while the health care assistants are learning.
- Extra time for the district nurses to review housebound patients that they visit.
- Protected time and funds for the pharmacist to introduce asthma reviews, education and self care plans and liaise with practice nurses.
- Time (and possibly training) for staff to implement, monitor and audit the project.

- Additional staffing hours may be needed initially – achieved by modifying the workload or extending the hours of existing staff or employing additional staff.

The outcomes might include:

> Either of Tools 9 or 12 will help to monitor progress

- better and more confident self care of asthma (P, A, R, T) by patients (**P**revent the condition, **A**wait resolution, use self care for **R**elief of symptoms, learn to **T**olerate symptoms) *see* Box 12.2, p. 153
- fewer episodes of admission in those who are using the programme (P, A, R, T)
- fewer inappropriate requests for GP appointments from patients with asthma that they could have avoided by doing self care (A, R, T)
- improvement in management of all zones of asthma by patients (A,R,T)
- fewer referrals to secondary care as there is better self care of asthma; concordance with treatment reduces the number and severity of attacks (P, A, R, T)
- no failures to identify and seek help appropriately for deterioration in asthma control (A, R, T)
- an active and useful support group for patients with asthma with expert input from those more experienced in its care (P, A, R, T)

How would you demonstrate that you have achieved your outcomes?

> Consider Tools 9 or 12 for reviewing outcomes

- Feedback (informal and formal) from patients about their self care of asthma, avoidance of triggers and confidence in monitoring their breathing patterns (P, A, R, T).
- Comparison of consultation rates for asthma at the practice before and after the project (P, A, R, T).
- Comparison of rates of review for asthma before and after the project (A, R, T).
- Comparison of the number of patients with a written self care action plan before and after the project (A, R, T).
- Comparison of emergency hospital admission rates for asthma before and after the project (P, A, R, T).
- Comparison of number and types of referrals to secondary care for asthma before and after the project (P, A, R, T).
- Self-rating and peer review of the effectiveness of education and use of written self care plans by nurses, pharmacist and GPs (P, A, R, T).
- Significant event audit of any failures to identify the necessity for medical input for deterioration of asthma control (A, R, T).

Illustrative patient pathway to self care: asthma

Table 12.1: Role and responsibilities checklist

For each task tick the box for each team member who has a role or responsibility – then note your role and responsibilities for the task.

Completed by _____

Task	Pharmacist	Practice nurses	Health care assistant	Patient	Reception team	GPs	Practice manager	Practice secretary	PCT	What are the roles and responsibilities?
Provision of information	✓	✓	✓	✓	✓	✓				Every person with asthma can be supplied with verbal and written information about asthma and self care
Written action plan	✓	✓	✓	✓		✓				Patients attending an asthma review receive a personalised written action plan that includes elements of self care
Significant event audit	✓	✓	✓	✓	✓	✓	✓			Any complaint or adverse outcome relating to patients consulting with asthma is examined
Audits of admissions, referrals, reviews and self care plans, etc	✓	✓	✓		✓	✓	✓	✓		Examination of the appropriateness of the admission or referral and the extent to which self care has been advocated and supported; discussion of the comparison of before and after reviews and plan; discussion and implementation of action for any change
Task 5 – you add										

Section 2 Self care for asthma

How big is the problem?

Eight million people in the UK have been diagnosed with asthma; 5.1 million are currently receiving treatment. On average 1400 people die from asthma each year in the UK. There were over 71 000 hospital admissions for asthma in the UK in 2001. An estimated 75% of hospital admissions for asthma are judged as avoidable, and 90% of deaths from asthma are preventable. Over 500 000 people with mild to moderate asthma report more than 25 asthma attacks in the previous 28 days. However, almost 50% of people with everyday asthma report that they are never or only occasionally asked by GPs how frequently they have had asthma attacks. Forty per cent are never or only occasionally asked about their symptoms more generally; 68% reported that their GP or practice nurse failed to enquire if their asthma had affected their ability to take part in any physical activities.[4]

Diagnosis

Ensure that patients being treated for asthma have their diagnosis confirmed. Diagnose asthma in adults by following the criteria taken from the USA and British guidelines on the care of asthma.[1,3,5] Symptoms can be episodic or variable and include cough, wheeze, shortness of breath and chest tightness. There are often no signs, but wheeze or increased breathing frequency may be present.

In addition, you may obtain a personal or family history of atopy, or symptoms may worsen following use of aspirin, NSAIDs drugs or beta blockers. People have often identified triggers e.g. pollen, dust, animals, exercise, viral infection, or chemical irritants. The pattern and severity of symptoms and exacerbations, e.g. following upper respiratory tract infections, may be characteristic.

Tests are helpful in distinguishing between hyperventilation, other lung conditions such as COPD and asthma (*see* Box 12.1).[1]

Box 12.1: Objective measurements

One of the following is diagnostic:

- more than 20% diurnal variation on at least three days a week in two successive weeks in peak flow diary
- forced expiratory volume in 1 second (FEV_1) increased by at least 15% (and 200 ml) after taking short acting $beta_2$ agonist (e.g. salbutamol 400 µg by metered dose inhaler in a spacer or 2.5 mg via nebuliser)
- FEV_1 increased by at least 15% (and 200 ml) after trial of steroid tablets (e.g. prednisolone 30 mg/day for 14 days)
- FEV_1 decreased by at least 15% after 6 minutes of exercise.

Initial education and advice

Patients given information at the time of diagnosis can make informed choices about their lifestyle, improving the self care of their asthma and reducing the burden on health care resources. A survey by Asthma UK showed that less than half the people with asthma learn how to recognise that their asthma is deteriorating or what to do if it does. Asthma UK, LungUSA and many other organisations provide written and web based information that patients can access.[6-8]

This information should accompany the assessment and provision of treatment at the relevant step of the guidelines.

Self care advice and guidance: take PART

Think of the range of advice and guidance about self care you might give to patients who consult you with asthma (*see* Box 12.2).

Box 12.2: Range of self care advice and guidance to give to patients

P *Prevention*: approximately 30–50% of the risk of developing asthma is caused by hereditary factors. Programmes to prevent asthma mainly focus on preventing triggers for asthma attacks. Colds cannot be prevented altogether, but annual immunisation can reduce the risk of influenza. Ensure that people with asthma understand the importance of avoiding influenza with relevant information and advice.[9,10]

Smoking and exposure to smoke are potent triggers for asthma. Ensure that everyone can receive information about and help with stopping smoking.[11] Non-smokers working in a smoky atmosphere e.g. in bars or clubs, should be having help from their employer in minimising their exposure.[12]

Isocyanates are a common cause of asthma at work. Spray painting, using adhesives, working in a foundry or making surface coatings are likely to involve exposure to isocyanates. Colophony present in adhesives, and dust from wood, grains, latex (beware latex gloves[13]) or animals may all be potent triggers for asthma. A list, frequently updated, is available from the Health and Safety Executive,[14] and liaison with personnel departments may be necessary to reduce or avoid exposure. The employer has a legal duty to reduce respiratory sensitisers at work.

Advice on breathing techniques may be helpful. Many patients with asthma have hyperventilation that may be a trigger for asthma, or may be mistaken for asthma.[15-17]

A *Awaiting* resolution of symptoms in asthma: this is only appropriate if patients are taking active steps to undertake self care of their symptoms. Self care plans should include time limits before contacting medical help.

R Plan self care for *relief* of symptoms: *see* outline in Box 12.3. Patients can obtain cards for completion, and much other information from Asthma UK.[5] The National Heart Lung and Blood Institute's *Practical Guide for the Diagnosis and Management of Asthma* also contains examples of self care plans.[3]

> **T** *Tolerance*: in people with mild asthma, progression to severe disease is rare. Although people with asthma lose lung function more rapidly than people without, progression is not as rapid as in smokers. People with chronic asthma can improve with treatment, but around 5% with severe disease respond poorly and are most at risk.[5] Help people to recognise that they should not *tolerate* disabling symptoms. Positive answers to the questions below should prompt a review of management:
> - have you had difficulty sleeping because of your asthma?
> - do you have asthma symptoms during the day?
> - have you found that your symptoms stop you doing everyday activities?

Action plans

Written personalised action plans as part of self care education have been shown to improve health outcomes for people with asthma.[18] Asthma UK established that patients preferred 'action plan' to 'self management plan' and most follow the concept of dividing the severity of symptoms and/or peak flow measurements into zones (*see* Boxes 12.1 and 12.3). Successful programmes include:[2,3]

- structured education with written personalised action plans
- specific advice about recognising the loss of asthma control by symptoms or peak flow readings or both. If peak flow readings are used, record the *actual figures* at which patients should take action. Expecting someone with deteriorating and frightening breathlessness to calculate a percentage of their previous best peak flow reading is unrealistic and counterproductive. Many people seem to have problems with percentages, but a calculator or computer aid can work the correct range out for them[18]
- action to take if the asthma deteriorates. This may include when to seek emergency help, starting on oral steroids (patients require an emergency supply at home), increasing inhaled steroids, or recommencing previous additional treatment as necessary for the level of symptoms or peak flow readings.

Personalise the patient's asthma care plan

Ask the patient to fill in the asthma care plan (as in Box 12.3) with their doctor or nurse.

Advise them to have a review every year at least to check that they are on the best treatment for their individual circumstances. Make sure that they can recognise their preventer and reliever medication, and know how to use them. Advise them to make sure that they have a spare inhaler of each type.

> **Box 12.3:** Action plan you can suggest to patients to optimise control of their asthma
>
> Management may be based on symptoms and/or peak flow readings completed in each box at the asthma review

Illustrative patient pathway to self care: asthma

Zone one/green zone (good control)
- You do not have, or only have very slight, symptoms in the day, or at night
- You can do all your normal activities without asthma symptoms
- Symptoms include: wheezing, coughing, shortness of breath, tightness of the chest
- Your best peak flow is
- Your peak flow is at or above (85% of your best)

Action plan
- Continue to take your usual asthma treatment
- Take your *preventer* medication every day even if you have no symptoms
- Take your *reliever* medication if you have symptoms

	Name	How much	When
Preventer 1			
Preventer 2			
Reliever			
Other			

If you are always at this level, discuss stepping down your medication at your next asthma clinic review.

Zone two/yellow zone (moderately worse)
Your asthma is worse and not well controlled if:

- you need to use your reliever inhaler more than once a day
- you have difficulty sleeping because of asthma
- your peak flow reading has fallen to between 70% to 80% of your best

Action plan
- Increase *preventer 1* to:
  Number of puffs/doses/day
- Increase *preventer 2* to:
  Number of puffs/doses/day

- Stay on this dose until you have had no symptoms for:
  Number of days:
- Then reduce your dose of *preventer* to that in Level one
- Continue to take your *reliever* as needed all the time
- Contact your doctor or nurse for advice if you do not improve in
  Number of days:

Your doctor or nurse will discuss your inhaler with you and perhaps check your technique. You may be started on a different medicine to control your symptoms.

If you are often at Level two, but do not need to contact your doctor or nurse each time, let them know at the next asthma review. You may need your medication increased or changed.

Zone three/yellow zone (much more severe)
Your asthma is much worse and poorly controlled if:

- you need to take your inhaler every four hours or even more often
- your symptoms are there all the time
- your peak flow reading is between 50% and 75% of your best

Action plan

- Take your *preventer* medication at the higher dose as listed in Level two
- Continue to take your *reliever* when you need it
- If you have been prescribed steroid tablets, take 5 mg prednisolone tablets *(number)* .... immediately and repeat each day for .... days or until your symptoms have improved or your peak flow has been at .... for two days
- Let your doctor or nurse know within 24 to 36 hours if you start a course of steroids *(delete if not required)*
- Let your doctor or nurse know within 36 to 48 hours if you are not improving after starting a course of steroids

If you are often at Level three but have not needed to contact the doctor or nurse, let them know at your next asthma review so that your usual medication can be adjusted.

Zone four/red zone (emergency)
Symptoms indicating an emergency are:

- your *reliever* is not helping
- your symptoms are getting worse (wheeze, cough, breathlessness, tight chest)
- you are too breathless to speak a sentence
- your peak flow reading is below

Action plan

- Sit up and loosen any tight clothing
- Take one puff/dose of your *reliever* every minute for five minutes or until symptoms improve
- If symptoms do not improve after five minutes, call 999

Structured educational asthma care plan

Trained health professionals usually deliver the reviews, education and action plans. Self care plans work best with appropriate prescribed asthma treatment within national guidelines.

Opportunities to rehearse the action plan occur when patients present with upper respiratory tract infections or other known triggers such as allergic rhinitis. An acute exacerbation offers the chance to go through what has been done already from the action plan, to reinforce the plan, or modify it if required.

Checklists for setting up a structured asthma programme (*see* Box 12.4) and for the content of an educational programme or discussion (*see* Box 12.5) have been derived from the SIGN guidelines.[2]

Box 12.4: A structured asthma care programme

1 Find the resources for written action plans and information leaflets. Non-promotional material is available from Asthma UK.[5]
2 Everyone on the team should give consistent advice.
3 Discuss how to deliver the programme, e.g. target those with most severe symptoms or everyone, integration of advice into usual care or into asthma clinics (or both), one-to-one consultations and/or in groups.
4 Tailor the education and advice to the individual needs of the patient. Some will want greater autonomy than others; and levels of ability to understand or to self care will vary.
5 Ensure that individuals know where to obtain further advice if the action plan does not provide the answer (a safety net).

Box 12.5: Possible content of an educational programme

1 The nature of the disease
2 What triggers exist for that patient and how they can be avoided or reduced
3 How asthma can be treated
4 Which effects of asthma the patient wants to control most
5 How to use the treatment
6 How to recognise the zones of deterioration
7 What barriers the patient has against recognising when the asthma is affecting them or against using treatment
8 Co-operation in designing the action plan to suit the needs of the patient
9 How to recognise the need for urgent help and how to obtain it

Tailor the information you give to the individual. Take into account the patient's educational level, reading ability, understanding, social and emotional factors, as well as their physical health. Take a look at the *Joining Up Self Care* initiative online.[19]

References

1. The British Thoracic Society, 17 Doughty Street, London EC1N 2PL www.brit-thoracic.org.uk
2. Scottish Intercollegiate Guidelines Network (SIGN), Royal College of Physicians, 9 Queen Street, Edinburgh EH2 1JQ www.sign.ac.uk
3. National Heart Lung and Blood Institute. *Practical Guide for the Diagnosis and Management of Asthma* www.nhlbi.nih.gov/health/prof/lung/asthma/practgde/practgdc.pdf
4. Tovey D (ed). *Clinical Evidence Concise (13)*. London: BMJ Publishing Group; 2005. www.besttreatments.co.uk/btuk/conditions/16360.html
5. www.asthma.org.uk
6. www.lungusa.org/site/pp.asp?c=dvLUK9OOE&b=38472
7. www.nlm.nih.gov/medlineplus/asthma.html
8. www.patient.co.uk/showdoc/23068771
9. www.asthma.org.uk
10. www.givingupsmoking.co.uk/nhs_sss
11. www.hse.gov.uk
12. www.hse.gov.uk/latex/primary.htm
13. www.hse.gov.uk/asthma
14. www.mja.com.au/public/issues/xmas98/bowler/refbody12
15. www.buteykobreathing.org
16. www.physiohypervent.org
17. Gibson PG, Powell H, Coughlan J et al. Self-management education and regular practitioner review for adults with asthma (Cochrane Review). *The Cochrane Library, Issue 3*. Oxford: Update Software; 2002. www.mrw.interscience.wiley.com/cochrane/clsysrev/articles/CD001117/frame.html
18. www.healthforums.com/topics/1,1258,home~8,00.html
19. www.wipp.nhs.uk

13

Illustrative patient pathway to self care: cough and colds
Gill Wakley

This chapter gives you an example of a practice team's approach to the self care of cough and colds.

Section 1 Self care for cough and colds

The start

We start with a patient's perspective. You could:

- work through the detailed scenario observing the sort of issues and discussion that the fictional practice team progress through here
- discuss how your team would respond to the patient story given here
- take an example case of a patient with a cough and cold from your own practice (anonymising the patient's identity in the team's discussion as appropriate).

If you do not know enough about the management of coughs and colds for completing the problem based learning, learn more about the range of self care support options and read through the clinical summary about cough and colds in the second section of this chapter, before you start the problem based learning exercise.

> **Patient's story 13.1**
> 'Tom is three years old and had only started at nursery a few weeks ago. He was hot, irritable and off his food for a couple of days over the weekend. He was coughing all the next night and kept waking up crying and asking for a drink, so I took him to the doctor. I was annoyed with the doctor who didn't seem to think Tom was ill at all and got us out of his room as quickly as he could. Mind you, Tom did seem much better than he had done in the night and was pulling all the drawers in the desk open and climbing on the couch. The doctor just listened to his chest and said to go on with the drinks and the paracetamol.
>
> I left it a couple of days and he was no better, so I took Tom back to see one of the other doctors. I had to wait ages to see that doctor and Tom embarrassed me by behaving badly. I told the doctor how ill he was at night, cough, cough, cough, until he was almost sick, even if he did perk up in the day. He just felt round Tom's neck, and then gave up examining him when Tom screamed and fought. The doctor wrote a prescription out for antibiotics. I

> wasn't sure, then, whether Tom really needed them. The doctor hadn't even listened to his chest again. Then after three days, Tom got diarrhoea, although he seemed better in himself. This time when I rang the practice, the receptionist suggested I talked to the health visitor. She was really sympathetic. She said she would ask the doctor and ring me back. When she did, she said to stop the antibiotics as they probably wouldn't make any difference to his cold, and told me lots of useful things to try with him. She said that I could always ring NHS Direct any time if I was worried about any of his symptoms or ask the pharmacist for advice. That made me feel more comfortable about managing his cough.'
>
> **Note**: the young patient and mother in this scenario had tried *awaiting* resolution of Tom's symptoms, *relief* of his symptoms with paracetamol and to some extent *tolerating* the symptoms.

The project team

> Consider Tool 11 on team building

You might want a team to discuss alternative self care support options for cough and colds as in this example to include:
- reception staff
- practice manager
- GPs
- practice nurses
- pharmacist
- health visitor
- patient representative.

You could use a checklist as in Table 13.1 to record who is involved and in what way.

Team discussion considering the patient story 13.1

> Consider Tools 1, 3, 4, 5, 6, 8 or 10 for your teamwork and discussions

In the scenario here, discussion between the fictional practice team members reveals:
- the pharmacist is not sure when the practice want adults or children referred to them. He usually refers people with green mucus, but has read that this does not always mean they need antibiotics. He has also read that cough medicines do not do much to help, but people seem to expect them

- the doctors manage colds and coughs inconsistently. The youngest doctor says he never gives antibiotics, the older ones say they usually do if the patient seems to expect it, or if they attend more than once. None of them spend much time explaining how patients might care for themselves, as the pressure of time when patients are seen urgently is too great
- the practice nurses are too busy seeing people with long term conditions in their chronic disease clinics to see any patients attending urgently with cough and colds, and feel that they are not competent to give advice or examine chests
- the health visitor feels that she is the expert here for advising parents. She has had training and lots of experience of advising mothers on childhood illness management. However, she is usually only in the practice on the day of the baby clinic and would find it difficult to liaise with the rest of the practice team on a more regular basis
- receptionists would like more guidance to prioritise those patients who need to see a doctor urgently
- the pharmacist usually delegates advice about cough and colds to the pharmacy assistants. No consistent policy has been agreed in the pharmacy. Neither have the GPs and local pharmacists agreed a policy for the treatment of cough, and the pharmacists are unaware of which patients the GPs feel should be seen
- the practice manager is concerned about the number of 'urgent extra' patients who have to be fitted into the appointments scheme. If these numbers could be reduced, more appointments bookable in advance could be released
- the patient representative feels that patients are made to feel a nuisance if they attend with cough and colds. He suggests that they should be able to talk to one of the doctors on the phone and receive antibiotics without being seen. The doctors are completely against this idea as, despite what they do in practice, they all agree antibiotics should not be used unless a secondary infection is suspected.

What you do next might include:

> Consider any of Tools 2, 3, 4, 5, 6, 7, 8, 9 or 10 for your action planning

- arrange a meeting for the members of the project team to look at ways that patients can be educated about prevention and following self care plans in relation to cough and colds as an example
- the practice manager and practice nurses agree to look at the workload. They need to decide if any of the work in chronic disease clinics can be done by other staff, or if more practice nurse time is needed, or if more training is required to extend their roles, or if a nurse practitioner could be trained or employed
- receptionists will receive training on using the NHS Direct algorithms,[1] to help them become more confident in advising patients on the most appropriate course of action – for example those ringing in with coughs or colds

- the patient representative will arrange for a patient advice leaflet and some posters to be piloted. The health visitor offers to obtain (or write) some leaflets for cough and colds, applicable to various age groups
- the doctors and nurses agree to meet with the practice or community pharmacist to examine the evidence about the treatment of cough and colds with antibiotics and other medication, and to draw up a policy so that patients receive consistent management from the GPs and local pharmacists. They will need to allow for patients to opt for symptomatic treatments that give them a temporary reduction in the discomfort of sore throat, even if there is no or limited evidence of any particular treatment providing a 'cure'
- the pharmacist will give patients a leaflet about overuse of antibiotics, and the practice will print out the patient information leaflet on Prodigy if the patient attends the practice.[2] The pharmacist might source the evidence, in addition to that presented in this chapter[3]
- the patient representative and practice manager will arrange some talks to the patient group. The GP agrees to talk about antibiotic use, and the health visitor and pharmacist will talk about self care
- doctors will use the patient information leaflets on Prodigy,[4,5] and the practice manager will ensure that all computers can print out patient information leaflets on the printers in the consulting rooms
- the practice manager and doctors discuss setting aside longer specific times for doctors to receive phone calls from patients, but this proves difficult and a decision is postponed until the 'extra urgent' patient demand is curtailed by other activity. The doctors feel that a nurse practitioner would be a better use of resources, to answer telephone queries about minor illnesses or undertake telephone triage, but might prove difficult to recruit
- the practice will approach the PCT for help with finding a nurse practitioner.

What extra resources might this require?

Consider either Tool 8, 10 or 17 for determining resource and skill needs

- Time for meetings and for training.
- Protected time for the practice manager to arrange meetings and training, monitor and support the introduction of the changes.
- Pharmacist, health visitor and GP time to talk to the patient group.
- Time for the GP and pharmacist to research material for clinical meetings.
- Time (and possibly training) for staff to implement, monitor and audit the project.
- Additional staffing hours may be needed initially – achieved by modifying the workload and hours of existing staff or employing additional staff. Also funding for a nurse practitioner or for one of the nurses to train as a nurse practitioner.

Illustrative patient pathway to self care: cough and colds

The outcomes might include:

> Either of Tools 9 or 12 will help to monitor progress

- better and more confident self care of cough and colds (P, A, R, T) (**P**revent the condition, **A**wait resolution, use self care for **R**elief of symptoms, learn to **T**olerate symptoms) *see* Box 13.1, p. 166
- more availability of suitable patient education and advice materials (P, A, R, T)
- fewer inappropriate requests for GP appointments from patients with cough and colds that could have been avoided by patients doing self care themselves (A, R, T)
- more appropriate consultations for complications of coughs and colds (A, R, T)
- no failures to identify and seek help appropriately for complications of coughs and colds (A, R, T)
- a trained nurse practitioner to take over the management and advice of minor illnesses and free up doctors for more complex illnesses (P, A, R, T).

How would you demonstrate that you have achieved your outcomes?

> Consider Tools 9 or 12 for reviewing outcomes

- Feedback (informal and formal) from patients about self care of colds and coughs.
- Comparison of consultation rates for colds and coughs at the practice before and after the project.
- Comparison of rates of advice given by the pharmacist before and after the project.
- Comparison of the number of patients, and the reasons for, referred by the pharmacist to the practice before and after the project.
- Self-rating and peer review of the effectiveness of education and use of information by nurses, pharmacist and GPs.
- An audit of minor ailment advice given over the telephone by GPs before and after the appointment of the nurse practitioner.
- Significant event audit of any failures to identify the necessity for medical input for complications of colds and coughs.

Table 13.1: Role and responsibilities checklist

For each task tick the box for each team member who has a role or responsibility – then note your role and responsibilities for the task.

Completed by _____

Task	Practice based or community pharmacist	Practice nurses	Health visitor	Patient	Reception team	GPs	Practice manager	PCT	What are the roles and responsibilities?
Provision of information (PART)	✓	✓	✓	✓	✓	✓		✓	Every person who attends with a cough and cold can be supplied with verbal and written information on self care of colds and cough
Significant event audit	✓	✓	✓	✓	✓	✓	✓		Any complaint or adverse outcome is examined in relation to patients consulting with cough or colds
Audits of attendances, referrals, etc	✓			(✓)	✓	✓	✓		Examination of the appropriateness of the patient referral from the pharmacist with cough or cold, extent to which self care has been advocated and supported; discussion of the comparison of before and after reviews and plan; discussion and implementation of action for any change
Task 4 – you add									
Task 5 – you add									

Section 2 Self care for cough and colds

How big is the problem?

Cough is the most common symptom presenting to medical practitioners.[6-8] Colds are common in children because they are often in close contact with each other in daycare centres and schools, and they are coming across the viruses for the first time. In families with children in school, the number of colds per child can be around 12 a year. Adults average about two to four colds a year, although the range varies widely. People older than 60 years of age generally have fewer than one cold a year.

What is it?

More than 200 viruses that can cause the common cold have been identified. The biggest offender, called the rhinovirus, causes up to 40% of colds and has 100 distinct types. Other important upper respiratory viruses include coronaviruses, adenovirus and respiratory syncytial virus.

Rhinoviruses have a well-established seasonal pattern, peaking after the summer months and again in spring. Other viruses tend to cause winter colds, which are usually more debilitating. Despite popular belief, there is little evidence that exposure to cold or rainy weather makes you more likely to catch a cold.[9]

Colds induced by different viruses differ primarily in their incubation period, ranging from 48–72 hours. Influenza virus produces consistently more severe symptoms in all age groups when compared to rhinovirus infection, and may be particularly debilitating in certain high risk patient groups.

People are most contagious for the first 2 to 3 days of a cold, and usually not contagious at all by days 7 to 10.

Symptoms and signs

Nasal discharge, a blocked nose, a sore throat, headache and cough are the most frequent complaints. Voice hoarseness, slightly sore eyes and feelings of pressure in the ears or sinuses also occur. The cough usually starts as the nasal discharge lessens. Body temperature is often increased especially in children. Night cough is an exhausting destroyer of sleep, especially for parents.

Babies may be irritable, have difficulty in feeding because of a blocked nose, and are more likely to have diarrhoea. Diagnosis in babies is more difficult, and raised body temperature may be the prominent symptom.

What else might it be?

Allergic or non-allergic rhinitis may present with similar symptoms, but usually without fever. Sore throat infections usually have more severe symptoms in the throat, but the disease spectrum overlaps. Influenza symptoms are usually much more severe, with systemic symptoms of high fever, sometimes with rigors, malaise and anorexia, and muscle pain being more prominent.

In children, a foreign body in the nose may cause one-sided discharge, or a cough, if the foreign body is inhaled or is in the external auditory meatus. In babies who are feeding poorly and appear ill, think about meningitis, septicaemia or pneumonia.

Self care advice and guidance: take PART

Think of the range of advice and guidance about self care you might give to patients who consult you with cough and colds (*see* Box 13.1).

Box 13.1: Range of self care advice and guidance for coughs and colds to give to patients and carers

P *Prevention*: cough is a symptom of a large number of illnesses. The commonest cause is an infection of the upper respiratory tract with other symptoms of fever, runny nose, sore throat, swollen neck glands, etc, usually labelled as a cold or 'flu-like illness. Look at Box 13.2 for suggestions about advice you can give to patients and the public about the prevention of colds and coughs.

A *Await* resolution of the symptoms: the NHS Direct algorithms on self care for coughing adults and coughing children give advice as to whether the cough requires treatment by a doctor or emergency services.[1] If the algorithm excludes a serious underlying cause, the cough is likely to be due to an upper respiratory tract infection (URTI). Uncertainty by both health professionals and the public about the natural course of coughs and colds may be partly responsible for the high consultation and repeat consultation rates and antibiotic use in primary care. A study of pre-school children with URTI symptoms found that only half had recovered by the tenth day and nine out of ten by the 25th day after symptoms started.[10] Many children still have nasal discharge and cough one week after presenting in a consultation in primary care, so that ideas about 'colds last a week' appear to be unrealistic.[11] Although fever may subside after a few days, symptoms due to mucus production (catarrh) may persist for 2–4 weeks in both children and adults. Decisions about the use of antibiotics should be based on the likely presence of bacterial infections, not by the length of time the illness has continued. Antibiotic treatment of people with URTI is not supported by current evidence from randomised trials.[12–14]

R Use self care for *relief* of symptoms: *see* outline in Box 13.3. Other advice on self care is given in the NHS Direct algorithm for colds and 'flu for children and adults.[1]

T Learn to *tolerate* symptoms: if symptoms continue without improvement, check with the NHS algorithm to ensure that symptoms have been evaluated correctly.[1] Persistent cough, or other symptoms may require medical examination or investigations.

Educate adults and parents about the simple measures to take to prevent coughs and colds (see Box 13.2) and to relieve the symptoms of straightforward colds and coughs (see Box 13.3), and give patients written information about self care. Avoid prescribing, as that tends to reinforce the tendency to attend for minor illnesses. If the patient expected an antibiotic, give a leaflet about antibiotic use. Ensure that adults and parents have access to information to make them more confident about diagnosing cough and colds and when they might need to seek other advice.[1] Information about prevention may be better targeted by posters and leaflets, or in response to queries.

Box 13.2: Advice to give patients and the public about prevention of colds and coughs

- Wash your hands frequently. Cold viruses are picked up on the hands and can be spread to the nose or eyes.
- Wash surfaces and articles used (especially toys) to avoid transfer of infection onto the hands.
- Exercise regularly.[15]
- Avoid smoke. This dries out the airway passages and paralyses the cilia (the minute hairs) that sweep out the mucus, dust and virus particles.
- A good mixed diet with plenty of fruit and vegetables will help to promote good general health.
- Complementary therapies may help. Echinacea, camomile, gingseng, and zinc have some limited evidence suggesting a beneficial effect,[15,16] but vitamin C in large doses has not been shown to be protective. Always check that herbal remedies will not affect other medicines or illnesses.

Persistent cough

If children or adults attend with a continuing cough this may be a symptom of a large number of conditions. The history is most likely to help with the diagnosis.[17] Adults who smoke are at risk of lung cancer and COPD. In asthma, persistent cough may be a symptom of poor control (see Chapter 12).

Complications of colds

Small babies under the age of three months are more likely to develop secondary bacterial infections. Young children may develop bronchiolitis, viral pneumonia and croup.[9] Adults over the age of 60 years are more likely to develop a lower respiratory tract infection, but the evidence for treatment with antibiotics is inconclusive. Most trials suggest that antibiotics shorten the course of bronchitis by about a day and are possibly associated with a higher risk of adverse effects.[18] A co-existing condition, such as COPD or diabetes, may change the balance of risks and benefits towards the use of antibiotics.

Otitis media occurs in around 2% of people with a cold and infection of the paranasal sinuses in around 0.5%.[19] Similar dilemmas exist about using antibiotics in these conditions. Antibiotics provide a small benefit for acute otitis media in children. As most cases will resolve spontaneously, this benefit must be weighed against possible adverse reactions.[20] Antibiotic treatment may play an important role in reducing the risk of mastoiditis in populations where it is more common.[21] The Cochrane review on treatments for maxillary sinusitis in adults found that antibiotics can help some people a bit but will not make a major difference to most.[21]

Box 13.3: Advice to give patients and the public about the relief of symptoms in coughs and colds

- Rest to allow the body time to heal itself.
- Increase your fluid intake by drinking water or fruit juices. This keeps the mucus (catarrh) watery and easier to cough up as well as relieving the sore throat.
- Avoid conditions that might make the cough worse. Smoke is very likely to make you worse. If you smoke, ask your pharmacist for advice about stopping.
- Very dry air or dust will also irritate the airways. Hanging wet towels on a radiator, or placing a bowl of water by a source of heat, or making the bathroom steamy, will all help to moisten the airways. Steam inhalations (for adults or older children) with a bowl of hot water may help to loosen sticky catarrh, but be careful with hot water, especially with children. Ask your pharmacist about adding aromatic preparations to the water.
- You can make your own drink with lemon and honey in warm water to relieve the cough and sore throat. Echinacea or vitamin C may be effective in shortening the length of time you have symptoms.
- Use extra pillows at night or, for younger children, prop up the whole of the top of the mattress on a folded blanket, to raise the head and reduce the amount of secretions dripping down the back of the throat.
- Ask the pharmacist for advice about paracetamol or ibuprofen for relief of pain and fever and about other medicines like cough linctus and decongestants. Check combination products to make sure you are not taking the same thing, like paracetamol, in several types and exceeding the recommended dose. Check that any medication does not interfere with other medicines you take.

Delayed prescription of antibiotics may help with the dilemma until the evidence is clearer about which patients may benefit most from antibiotics for secondary infections or complications.[22]

References

1. www.nhsdirect.nhs.uk
2. Schroeder K and Fahey T. Over-the-counter medications for acute cough in children and adults in ambulatory settings (Cochrane Review). *The Cochrane Library, Issue 4.* Oxford: Update Software; 2004.

3   *Why no Antibiotic?* (Patient information leaflet) www.prodigy.nhs.uk/ProdigyKnowledge/PatientInformation/Content/pils/PL212.htm

4   Common cold advice leaflet for adults www.prodigy.nhs.uk/ProdigyKnowledge/PatientInformation/Content/pils/PL294.htm

5   Common cold advice leaflet for children www.prodigy.nhs.uk/ProdigyKnowledge/PatientInformation/Content/pils/PL43.htm

6   Cherry DK, Burt CW and Woodwell DA. National Ambulatory Medical Care Survey: 2001 summary. *Advance Data.* 2003; **337:** 1–44.

7   Morice AH. Epidemiology of cough. *Pulmonary Pharmacology and Therapeutics.* 2002; **15:** 253–9.

8   www.cdc.gov

9   Prodigy guidance on common cold. www.prodigy.nhs.uk

10 Hay AD, Wilson A, Fahey T and Peters TJ. The duration of acute cough in pre-school children presenting to primary care: a prospective cohort study. *Family Practice.* 2003; **20:** 696–705.

11 Hay AD and Wilson AD. The natural history of acute cough in children aged 0–4 years in primary care: a systematic review. *British Journal of General Practice.* 2002; **52:** 401–9.

12 Fahey T, Stocks N and Thomas T. Systematic review of the treatment of upper respiratory tract infection. *Archives of Disease in Childhood.* 1998; **79:** 225–30.

13 www.aafp.org/afp/981015ap/dowell.html

14 Aroll B and Kenealy T. Antibiotics for the common cold and acute purulent rhinitis (Cochrane Review). *The Cochrane Library, Issue 4.* Oxford: Update Software; 2003.

15 Ernst E (ed). *The Desktop Guide to Complementary and Alternative Medicine: an evidence based approach.* London: Harcourt Publishers; 2001.

16 Prasad AS, Fitzgerald JT, Bao B, Beck FW and Chandrasekar PH. Duration of symptoms and plasma cytokine levels in patients with the common cold treated with zinc acetate. A randomized, double-blind, placebo-controlled trial. *Annals of Internal Medicine.* 2000; **133:** 302–3.

17 Hopcroft K, Forte V. *Symptom Sorter.* Oxford: Radcliffe Medical Press; 1999.

18 Fahey T, Smucny J, Becker L and Glazier R. Antibiotics for acute bronchitis (Cochrane Review). *The Cochrane Library, Issue 4.* Oxford: Update Software; 2004.

19 www.nntonline.net/ebm/newsletter/200210/200210.asp

20 Glasziou PP, Del Mar CB, Sanders SL and Hayem M. Antibiotics for acute otitis media in children (Cochrane Review). *The Cochrane Library, Issue 1.* Oxford: Update Software; 2004.

21 Williams JW, Aguilar C, Cornell J *et al.* Antibiotics for acute maxillary sinusitis. *The Cochrane Library, Issue 2.* Oxford: Update Software; 2003.

22 Arroll B, Kenealy T, Goodyear-Smith F and Kerse N. Delayed prescriptions (editorial). *British Medical Journal.* 2003; **327:** 1361–2. http://bmj.bmjjournals.com/cgi/content/full/327/7428/1361

Part 3

Tools to help you plan and support self care
Ruth Chambers and Gill Wakley

These 21 tools give you some tried and tested techniques to help you devise your strategy and action plan to implement a self care culture. Turn back to Figures 3.1 and 4.1 to see how these tools fit in to the various stages you will work through to evolve and establish a culture of supporting self care in your PCT or practice. The illustrative patient pathways of Chapters 10–13 flagged up the various tools too at pertinent points.

Tool 1 Force-field analysis
Tool 2 Devising your PCT/practice strategy and action plan to establish a new culture of promoting and supporting self care (Devising strategy and action plan)
Tool 3 Strengths, weaknesses, opportunities and threats (SWOT) analysis (SWOT)
Tool 4 The basic planning process: taking account of political, economic, sociological and technological factors (PEST)
Tool 5 The Gap model
Tool 6 Plan, do, study, act (PDSA) model for improvement
Tool 7 Timetable tasks with a Gantt chart
Tool 8 Infrastructure and resource matrix
Tool 9 Undertake an audit of how well established support for self care is in your practice
Tool 10 Training needs analysis
Tool 11 How well is your team functioning? (Team function checklist)
Tool 12 Significant event audit
Tool 13 PART/workload assessment
Tool 14 Moving through change
Tool 15 Keep a reflective learning log
Tool 16 Reduce time pressures at work
Tool 17 Check out whether supporting self care is a priority for your practice and whether the way in which you plan to learn about it is appropriate (Priority check list)
Tool 18 Draw up a personal map of support mechanisms in your life (Personal support mapping)
Tool 19 Assess your consultation skills and style (Consultation content scale)
Tool 20 Determine your consulting style (Consulting style scale)
Tool 21 Self care consultation style: encouraging, guiding and supporting patients to adopt self care (Self care aware consulting style)

Tool 1

Force-field analysis

This technique gives you:
- a way of diagnosing a situation
- a means of planning for change
- a way of implementing a change strategy and programme.

With this approach, there will be one set of influences and pressures *pushing for a change* and a different set *pushing to keep things as they are*.

- Driving forces are factors that indicate instability and an openness towards change. They are therefore *positive* forces for change.
- Restraining forces are those that promote stability and maintain the status quo: indicating, therefore, *resistance* to change.

In effect any situation is really a state of 'dynamic equilibrium' between these two sets of forces. Change will occur when the interplay of various forces and influences at play in a particular situation alters. When you change the net effect of the influences involved, the situation will realign itself into a new 'dynamic equilibrium'. Rather than trying to force others to change their views, you should try to reduce some of their reasons for resisting change, so re-balancing the situation, enabling change to occur. Just pushing harder and harder for what you want to happen, may just make people dig their heels in and resist.

With a force-field analysis approach the interconnections between different influences and forces are more easily seen, and can help you decide which influences to work on first.

Draw up a force-field analysis of the culture of self care in your PCT or practice

Why you should use this

To help people identify and focus down on the positive and negative forces in the development of a self care culture and gain an overview of the weighting of these factors.

When to use this

In a PCT or practice planning day or team meeting – as an individual or preferably working in a group.

What to do

Draw a horizontal or vertical line in the middle of a sheet of paper. Label one side 'positive' and the other side 'negative'. Draw arrows to represent individual positive drivers that motivate you and the PCT/practice team on one side of the line, and negative factors that demotivate you on the other side of the line. The chunkiness and length of the arrows should represent the extent of the influence; so, a short, narrow arrow will indicate that the positive or negative factor has a minor influence, and a long, wide arrow indicates a major effect.

Take an overview of the force-field and consider if you are content with things as they are, or can think of ways to boost the positive side and minimise the negative factors. You can do this part of the exercise on your own, with a peer or a small group, or with a mentor, or trainer from the PCT.

How it works (insight)

You realise whether a known influence in your life is a positive or negative factor. For instance you may realise upon reflection that you had assumed that reducing your workload was the main positive motivator. But really, the wish to empower patients to lead healthier lives through self care is your main motivator, giving added benefit of improving your job satisfaction.

Whom to engage

The exercise is suitable for anyone and everyone in the PCT/practice team who has contact with patients or has a public health or health promotion or public involvement role. Include local community pharmacists too to gain a wider perspective and collaboration.

How much time you should allow

Up to an hour with ensuing discussion. Longer for subsequent action planning.

What a facilitator should do

Urge participants to subsequent action.

What to do next

Make a personal or organisational action plan to boost the positive factors in establishing a self care culture and minimise arrows on the negative side.

What makes it work better

Get someone who knows the context well to review the force-field analysis and comment on any blind spots and whether positive and negative influences are in proportion. This might be someone from another general practice who is already promoting and supporting self care there.

What can go wrong

People perpetuate their own misconceptions – and use the force-field analysis diagram to reinforce their negative or resistant behaviour in a pseudo-scientific way.

Force-field analysis

An example of a force-field analysis is shown in Box T1.1.

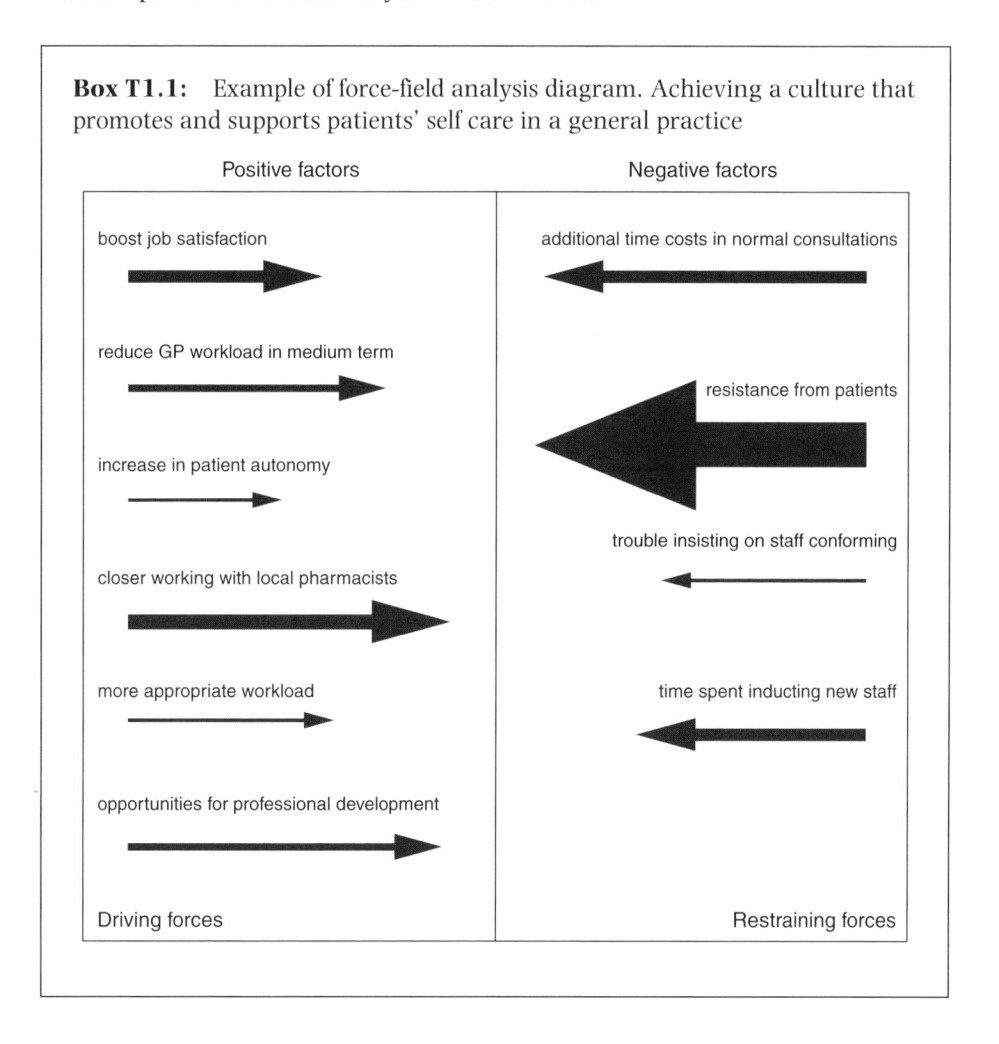

Box T1.1: Example of force-field analysis diagram. Achieving a culture that promotes and supports patients' self care in a general practice

Positive factors	Negative factors
boost job satisfaction →	← additional time costs in normal consultations
reduce GP workload in medium term →	← resistance from patients
increase in patient autonomy →	← trouble insisting on staff conforming
closer working with local pharmacists →	← time spent inducting new staff
more appropriate workload →	
opportunities for professional development →	
Driving forces	Restraining forces

Tool 2

Devising your PCT/practice strategy and action plan to establish a new culture of promoting and supporting self care

Creating a strategy and statement of intent

The development of any strategy requires commitment and action from the organisation's leadership, to give it authority. You want to develop an environment where self care by patients is consistently valued and encouraged by all the workforce. A good strategy will ensure that an integrated self care support resource is developed and patients are provided with a wide range of self care support options to choose from.

This tool will offer a framework for senior managers and key stakeholders to identify which of the success criteria they already have or are working towards. Do it at a standard planning meeting or with a dedicated working group focused on the promotion and support of self care.

Part 1: define your initial aims and people's ideas about their contributions

Why you should do this

This activity focuses on what people hope to achieve, and parts they need to play.

When to use this

Useful at the beginning of a session to construct an action plan to introduce the work that needs to be covered.

What to do

Give everyone a sheet of flip chart paper. Ask them to draw a line across the middle about half-way down. Head the top section 'Aims', the lower half 'Contributions'. Ask them to list their own aims for the session and what they will contribute to the session to achieve them. Fix the sheets to the wall. Encourage everyone to read other people's sheets.

Alternatively, get each person to do a similar task before they come to the planning meeting. Then use their completed paperwork to kickstart discussions.

Devising your PCT/practice strategy and action plan

Table T2.1: Checklist for what makes up a strategy and statement of intent

	Criteria – you have:	Where are we now?	Your action
1	a strategy and statement of intent specifically constructed with promotion of self care and development of an integrated self care support resource at the centre		
2	specific standards relating to funding, resources, protected time, training etc and other minimum requirements – applied to everyone involved in promoting and supporting self care		
3	defined the affordable vision		
4	representatives of the workforce involved in the development of policies and implementation plans		
5	described the training plan to match the strategy and affordable vision		
6	communicated the strategy, statement of intent and implementation plan throughout the PCT/practice		
7	evaluation methods developed to measure effectiveness, outcomes and contribution to organisational objectives		

How it works (insight)

People will 'own' what they've written, and become clearer about why they are attending the meeting. They define their role and can see that they need to be actively involved, not just passive observers.

Whom to engage

This is a useful start for any planning group.

How much time you should allow
Thirty minutes if the exercise is used as a simple checklist and up to three hours if used as part of a developmental event.

What a facilitator should do
Keep time, wander around encouraging anyone who is not getting started.

What to do next
The two exercises which follow, continue and refine this activity.

What makes it work better
People with a clear idea what they want from attending, and what they can do to achieve their aims – so provide some pre-reading matter.

What can go wrong
- Participants who have been sent rather than wanting to attend for themselves, and make a reluctant input to the action plan.
- Participants who have no clear idea what they want or what they can contribute to promoting and supporting self care.

Part 2: refining the aims into objectives; using the contributions

Why you should do this
It shows that you are responding to the stated aims and examining how (and if) they could be met by using the contributions of the team members.

What to do
Review the sheets of the previous exercise (Part 1) and identify some general categories. Write these as headings on a flip chart or PowerPoint slide.

Ask each person to stand by their sheet and in turn to read out one aim. Ask the group to provide an objective that would meet the aim, and into which category it would fit, then ask what contributions from team members would help it to be realised. Write the objectives in one colour, the contributions in another. Add in any activities already planned that meet the objectives. You will need a 'miscellaneous' category for those that do not fit neatly into any one category.

Leave the aims and objectives displayed for you and the participants to check out whether they are being met (be prepared to modify what you do accordingly!).

Devising your PCT/practice strategy and action plan

How it works (insight)
People can judge whether their aims are reasonable or over-ambitious and unlikely to be met. They can recognise where their own contributions can assist with setting and meeting objectives, and where they fit in with the activities planned.

Whom to engage
The aims and contributions need to have been collected first.

How much time you should allow
Discussion usually takes about 40–60 minutes.

What a facilitator should do
Encourage discussion of aims and contributions. Allow new contributions to be offered, and modify the aims if people realise they are unrealistic. Try to categorise the aims and objectives as clearly as possible.

What to do next
You might use the following exercise (Part 3).

What makes it work better
- People who are prepared to be flexible about what they have written down and are prepared to be responsible for their own learning.
- Team members who have similar aims.

What can go wrong
- People who cannot (or will not) recognise that their aims are unrealistic, or who cannot see that they could make any contribution towards meeting them.
- Widely different aims among the participants.

Part 3: setting priorities

Why you should do this
Team members must recognise that not all their aspirations are possible with competing pressures, so they need to set priorities.

When to use this
You might use this for any suggested activity where there are a large number of objectives, not all of which can be met within the resources available or timetable suggested.

What to do

List objectives on the flip chart and give a letter of the alphabet (A, B, C, etc) to the objectives obtained. Ask each participant to rate each objective from 1–20 and write the rating by the letter without conferring. Explain that it is alright to allocate the total of '20' marks to one item, and to rate another as 'zero', or to split the marks more equally. Ask each group member to give you their ratings and write them alongside the objectives. Add up the total rating for each objective.

If there are objectives with widely different ratings, ask the person who gave it a high rating to explain why, and the person who gave it a low rating to reply. Allow a general discussion for each objective with different ratings.

How it works (insight)

It can be surprising for some people to discover that items they rated as important were not so to others. It emphasises the need to explore other people's views of what is important and take their views into account when setting out a programme of work.

Whom to engage

Preferably all those who have contributed so far; or a smaller working group otherwise, with or without external colleagues.

How much time you should allow

This depends on the degree of disagreement. If ratings are similar, it will take about half an hour, but twice that if items are hotly argued over.

What a facilitator should do

Keep the peace – do not allow feelings to become too heated in defence of someone's pet idea. Move the discussion on fairly briskly to avoid spending all the time discussing just a few of the points.

What to do next

Use the priority ratings to hand over specific objectives to small development groups – allocate the items they rated highly to those most interested. Modify the content of the activities to make them more relevant to the highly rated objectives. Offer to set up further groups to meet objectives that cannot be covered in the time available.

What makes it work better

Differences in the participants' views – this is more likely if they come from different health or management disciplines.

What can go wrong

- Everyone agrees on the priorities and there is little or no discussion.
- A few people become upset that their objectives are not rated highly by others.

Tool 3

Strengths, weaknesses, opportunities and threats (SWOT) analysis

Why you should use this

This tool can be used to analyse the capability of your PCT or practice team now and in the future, in planning to promote and support self care. It identifies promoters and resistors to change within four key dimensions.

When to use this

When you are taking stock of an issue or situation, before putting together your plan to address it and improve matters.

What to do

Define the purpose of the exercise.

Everyone should group around a single flip chart to be able to see the four quadrants at once:

Strengths	Weaknesses
Opportunities	Threats

Each section is then completed through discussion with questions that explore your perceptions of the challenge in establishing and promoting an integrated self care support resource and the environmental influences that can help or hinder. For example:

1 *strengths*: what are we good at already (e.g. promotion/education on healthy lifestyles)?
2 *weaknesses*: what are we bad at (e.g. maybe poor at encouraging patients who are housebound or seriously ill to consider self care as an option)?
3 *opportunities*: what's around the corner that could be useful? What is new, and is it good for us?
4 *threats*: what could be a threat to our success? What's new and is it bad for us?

Once you have completed all four quadrants of the SWOT analysis you should consider:

- how can you maximise and extend the strengths identified?
- how can you minimise or overcome the weaknesses?
- how can you make use of the opportunities?
- how can you avoid the threats or counter their effects?

How it works (insight)

It captures everyone's views so that you get all perspectives. Because of the informal atmosphere, certain individuals are unlikely to dominate, and completing the SWOT can be a reasonably democratic process.

Whom to engage

Everyone involved in the issue or situation under discussion, and whose support and engagement are needed to draw on the strengths and opportunities and combat weaknesses and threats.

How much time you should allow

At least an hour for undertaking the SWOT analysis, completing the lists in each quadrant, and making preliminary conclusions about next steps.

What a facilitator should do

Engage the people who need to be present to complete the SWOT and ensuing action plan, set the scene, explain the nature of the exercise. Agree the specific purpose of the exercise and subsequent work.

What to do next

Write up the SWOT analysis and preliminary conclusions and any action plan. Ask key participants to revise the document. Be a link between completion of the SWOT and evolution of the action plan. Ensure the action plan is do-able – and help to take it forward across the PCT/practice according to the purpose.

What makes it work better

- Involvement of senior people in the PCT/practice planning the SWOT analysis and how it fits with strategy, policy and action.
- An informal and friendly environment where everyone feels that their views are valued so that they contribute whatever their role.

What can go wrong

The SWOT analysis being undertaken in a 'vacuum' so that the material produced is not used afterwards and little happens as a result.

Tool 4

The basic planning process: taking account of political, economic, sociological and technological (PEST) factors

Environmental perspectives include:
- political
- economic
- sociological
- technological factors.

Why you should use this
A PEST analysis focuses on factors external to the PCT or practice allowing analysis of drivers that may or may not be within the organisation's control. A PEST analysis should be carried out in the context of the broader picture – the climate in which the PCT/practice operates.

When to use this
For defining the PCT's or practice's future purpose – in this instance, supporting self care and developing an integrated resource for self care. Or as a template for a team-building event over a half/whole day.

What to do
There are three stages in the planning process:
- Stage 1: establish the organisation's current position
- Stage 2: define where the organisation wants to be (1–3 years)
- Stage 3: map the gap by identifying what you need to get there.

Discuss the political, economic, sociological and technological factors that influence your PCT's/practice's aims and objectives:

Political	Economic
Sociological	**Technological**

How it works (insight)

Start with an assessment of where the PCT/practice is currently – in relation to promoting self care and developing an integrated resource to support self care; what influences this aim and what factors affect it. So the PEST analysis should reflect the perspectives and issues of other healthcare providers, patient groups and target population and the current local situation (politically and in terms of the level of social capital). It should draw on profiles, audits and surveys that are relevant.

Whom to engage

This could be the executive teams in the PCT or key personnel in a practice team.

How much time you should allow

Two hours to a whole day (dependent on application and target group).

What a facilitator should do

Engage the people who need to be present to complete the PEST analysis and ensuing action plan, set the scene, explain the nature of the exercise. Encourage those taking part to agree the specific purpose and subsequent work.

What to do next

Write up the PEST analysis and preliminary conclusions and any action plan. Ask key participants to revise the document. Be a link between completion of the PEST and evolution of the action plan. Ensure the action plan is do-able – and help to take it forward across the PCT/practice and with external stakeholders, according to the purpose.

What makes it work better
- Involvement of senior people in the PCT/practice planning, and completion of the PEST analysis ensuring it fits with strategy, policy and action.
- An informal and friendly environment where everyone feels that their views are valued so that they can contribute, whatever their role in the organisation.
- Engagement and contributions from the external parties whose views are key to the discussion of political, economic, sociological and technical perspectives relevant to the promotion and development of self care support.

What can go wrong
- The PEST analysis being undertaken in a 'vacuum' so that the material produced is not used afterwards and little happens as a result
- Too few 'outsiders' being involved, so that the PCT/practice do not appreciate others' perspectives of their plans.

Tool 5

The gap model

Why you should use this

It helps people to look at and discuss the size and nature of the gap between their current situation and where they want to be by a defined time in the future. It helps to plan how to minimise or close the gap.

When to use this

Before planning changes to services.

What to do

An outline gap analysis:
   Figure T5.1 represents what has to be done to close the gap.

1. *Where we are now*: assess what is important to your situation and relevant to the changes you want to make.
2. *Define the desired future*: build up a complete picture to give everyone the clearest indication of what standards are to be achieved.
3. *Define the gap*: compare 1 and 2 and specify the major differences between the current picture and desired future position. Differences identified indicate the scope and detail of the changes that need to take place to reach the desired position.

How it works (insight)

The gap forms the basis for a programme of change – in relation to establishing a culture of promoting patients' self care and developing an integrated resource to support self care. The actual programme of change is determined by the various gaps identified.

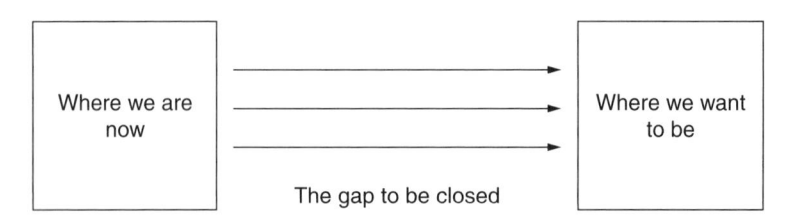

Figure T5.1: Closing the gap.

Whom to engage
People who are going on to draw up plans for services or setting priorities or categories for promoting and supporting self care, within a budget or available resources.

How much time you should allow
Allow 45–60 minutes for discussion.

What a facilitator should do
Prevent the discussion becoming personalised or too narrow. Keep the time and encourage discussion and an action-orientated approach.

What to do next
Take up the suggestions made if they are practical, or explain why you cannot if not. Gain commitment for the action plan – who will do what, when and how.

What makes it work better
- Participants who have previous experience of action planning work and reflective practice – to consider the many contributory factors to the present situation.
- People with creative ideas about how to close the gap.

What can go wrong
Participants do not take the task seriously and propose unrealistic ideas to close the gap.

Tool 6

Plan, do, study, act (PDSA) model for improvement

Why you should use this
To develop, test and implement changes that lead to improvement.

When to use this
When your team needs to set clear and focused goals in relation to promoting and supporting self care.

What to do
The model for improvement is represented in Figure T6.1.
The aims statement should:

- be consistent with national and local targets, plans and frameworks (such as the QOF or NSFs)
- be bold in its aspirations
- have clear numerical targets.

There are four stages to a PDSA cycle:

- *plan*: plan the change to be tested or implemented
- *do*: carry out the test or change
- *study*: study data before and after the change and reflect on what was learnt
- *act*: plan the next change cycle or plan implementation.

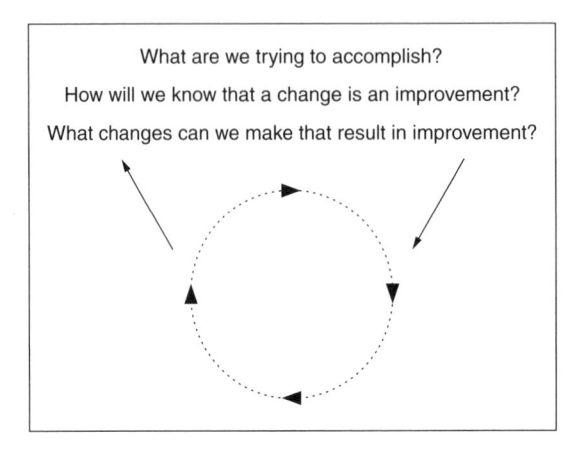

What are we trying to accomplish?
How will we know that a change is an improvement?
What changes can we make that result in improvement?

Figure T6.1: The model for improvement.

Plan, do, study, act (PDSA) model for improvement

How it works (insight)

A PDSA cycle involves testing improvement ideas on a small scale before introducing the change. By building on the learning from the test cycles in a structured and incremental way, a new idea can be implemented with greater chance of success. Barriers to change are often reduced when different people are involved in trying something out on a small scale before implementation.

Whom to engage

Use this exercise for small mixed groups of people. For example an inter-professional group might consider the roles, responsibilities or experiences of the different professions involved in promoting and supporting self care; a practice team might tackle motivating people to adopt self care or creating resources for team members who are supporting self care.

How much time you should allow

Allow an hour for discussion and planning. Re-convene the working group at two more stages in the PDSA process, allowing at least an hour at each meeting.

What a facilitator should do

Explain the time and effort commitment to everyone at the initial meeting. Arrange two more meeting dates to follow the planning session that everyone can make – to study the data after the piloted change and review how you will act; then at a later date to review the change you've made and determine how successful it is and what else needs doing.

What to do next

Collect baseline data. Formulate a detailed action plan at a planning session so everyone knows how to play their part in the do stage. Link with key players throughout, communicating progress to all involved.

What makes it work better

- Commitment from senior people in the PCT or practice.
- Protected time for those involved to *do* the plan, *study* the progress and take further *action*.

What can go wrong

- Big ideas without the resources to take the planned change forward.
- A 'project' mentality so that the change does not settle into being part of everyone's core work.

An improvement cycle report template is shown in Table T6.1.

Table T6.1: Improvement cycle report template (as derived from Lambeth, Southwark and Lewisham PCTs)

Objective:		Your response
Plan	• What exactly will you do?	
	• Who will be involved and how?	
	• When will it take place?	
	• Where will it take place?	
	• What will you measure?	
	• What do you predict will happen?	
Do	• Implement the plan and record:	
	– what was actually done and when	
	– any unexpected observations or problems	
	• Collate and begin to analyse data	
Study	• What were the results?	
	• Did they differ from your expectations (if so, how/why)?	
	• What have you learnt from this cycle?	
Act	• What action will you now take to:	
	– refine your improvement idea and re-test it or	
	– implement it and embed the change or	
	– reject the idea and prepare to test a new one?	

Tool 7

Timetable tasks with a Gantt chart

Why you should use this
To enable you to make a timetabled plan for improving the management of a current service you provide or to set up a new resource on supporting self care in the local community or to your patients.

When to use this
For an interactive workshop or small group work with individuals from different organisations or the same organisation (e.g. a practice, a PCT).

What to do
- *Stage 1*: everyone contributes all the aspects of organisational management needed to set up a new service (e.g. an integrated resource to support self care). These are captured on a flip chart. When the ideas have dried up, the flip chart papers are displayed.
- *Stage 2*: participants fix the order that jobs should be tackled to achieve a well organised and managed service, as a Gantt chart (*see* Table T7.1).
- *Stage 3*: compare Gantt charts if more than one. Look at the range and type of factors considered, and the timing of each aspect. Add new features to the Gantt chart and change the timing as appropriate.
- *Stage 4*: the lead reflects on the priorities for organisational management of the promotion of self care and of setting up a new service or resource to support self care.
- *Stage 5*: final review of individual Gantt chart(s) and decide if you wish to extend the contents to add new factors or change the timing of activities.

How it works (insight)
The individuals should move along a spectrum of learning about organisational management from Stage 2 to Stage 4 when they can listen to the lead and consider where their plans are lacking, to Stage 5 when discussion with others addresses gaps and there is a final review.

The Gantt chart is a useful planning aid that forces the PCT or practice team to identify all the activities that will be involved at any particular time, to ensure that there are sufficient resources.

Whom to engage
This is an exercise for novices in organisational management.

How much time you should allow

At least an hour to allow time for discussion, but it depends on how complex the setting up of the new culture of self care will be.

What a facilitator should do

Demonstrate how to make up a Gantt chart – show that it can be produced on a computer or by drawing by hand.

What to do next

Encourage participants to put their new-found knowledge into practice by pursuing their timetabled activity plan.

What makes it work better

- A lead who is content to stand back and let the participants work through their planning stages.
- Ask people to describe a few current problems with self care. Test out whether the new plan is designed to proactively deal with those particular problems.

What can go wrong

- Participants may be reluctant to co-operate.
- Non-managers (e.g. clinicians) are not interested because they do not consider that organisational management is their responsibility.

An example of a Gantt chart is given in Table T7.1.

Timetable tasks with a Gantt chart

Table T7.1: Example of a Gantt chart – promoting self care support across a PCT or practice

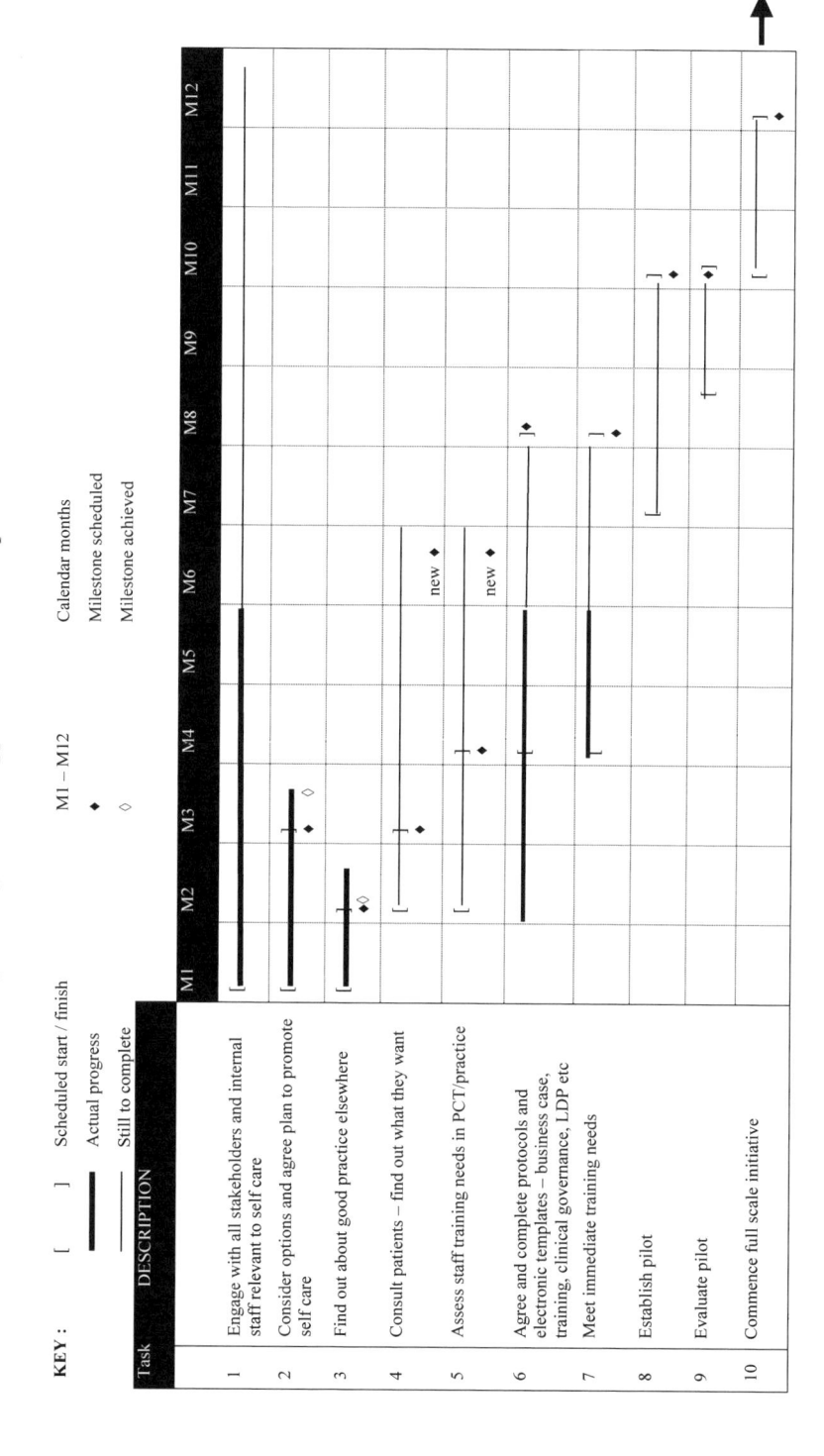

KEY:
- [ ] Scheduled start / finish
- ▬ Actual progress
- ─── Still to complete
- M1 – M12 Calendar months
- ◆ Milestone scheduled
- ◇ Milestone achieved

Task	DESCRIPTION	M1	M2	M3	M4	M5	M6	M7	M8	M9	M10	M11	M12
1	Engage with all stakeholders and internal staff relevant to self care												
2	Consider options and agree plan to promote self care												
3	Find out about good practice elsewhere												
4	Consult patients – find out what they want												
5	Assess staff training needs in PCT/practice						new						
6	Agree and complete protocols and electronic templates – business case, training, clinical governance, LDP etc						new						
7	Meet immediate training needs												
8	Establish pilot												
9	Evaluate pilot												
10	Commence full scale initiative												

Tool 8

Infrastructure and resource matrix

Why you should use this
To assess the readiness of your organisation's infrastructure in the development of self care support. The matrix should help you to plot gaps in resource availability.

When to use this
While taking stock of your baseline resources in the preliminary stages of evolving an action plan for a new initiative such as promoting and supporting self care.

What to do
Study Table T8.1 and plot your PCT/practice's resources by ticking where there are identified resources available and making a cross where there are none in the matrix in Table T8.2.

How it works (insight)
Identifying gaps in infrastructure or resources enables you (as a PCT/practice) to build an action plan of the next steps to promoting and supporting self care.

Whom to engage
This exercise can be used by teams, PCT directorate or the practice as a whole, to identify resource needs.

How much time you should allow
A one hour discussion with homework by some individuals afterwards to fill in the gaps.

What a facilitator should do
Describe the task to be completed before participants gather to discuss resources. Encourage people to come prepared with information about current resources. Ensure someone is nominated to receive follow-on information.

What to do next
Feed the completed table into the action planning process.

Infrastructure and resource matrix

Table T8.1: Resource matrix

Symbol	Infrastructure/resource	Explanation
	Documentation	Policy, protocols, standards, operating procedures, etc
	Location	Physical location, available space, training facilities etc
	Money	Protected/identified funding, budgets, bids, grants etc
	Expertise	Skills, knowledge, capability, competence within or without the organisation. Training and education provision
	People	Appropriately trained and available staff, staff hours, coverage for training etc
	Materials	Equipment, books, training resources, supplies, provisions etc
	Information technology	Hardware, software, networks, internet capability, library facilities, knowledge management systems
	Communication	e.g. newsletter, team briefing, user involvement, community, media and press
	Planning	Planning mechanisms, planning groups, project management capability, strategic planning meetings, links to Department of Health policies

What makes it work better
The right people completing the table so that accurate information and reasonable guesstimates are contributed.

What can go wrong
Information about resources is inaccurate, predictions are unrealistic, assumptions are made and any guesstimates are too low, so participants underestimate the need for future resources for the new initiative to be put into place, piloted and succeed.

Table T8.2: Matrix – take stock of the resources you will need for supporting self care in your PCT/practice

	Resources								
Infrastructure									
Education policy, has reference to self care									
Education/training budget re promoting and supporting self care									
Training needs analysis process									
Induction programme for new staff									
Library facilities – staff/patients									
Literature for promoting and supporting self care (relevant languages)									
Health promotional aids (visual, audio)									
Communication system, for consistent approach by PCT/practice team									
Protected time for starting/doing new initiatives									
Risk management processes									
Partnership learning with other PCT/practice									
Other (you add rows you need):									

Please note that all columns will be appropriate for each aspect of infrastructure.

Tool 9

Undertake an audit of how well established support for self care is in your practice

Why you should use this

Clinical audit helps you to review the way your practice organisation works as a whole – and make improvements. It will help you to improve the quality of self care support you provide.

When to use this

You might audit:

- the range of self care support provided
  - by the doctor/nurse/practice pharmacist/health care assistant/reception staff/practice systems
  - whether it concerns prevention and treatment for common minor conditions and long term conditions e.g. information provision (verbal/printed/web based/noticeboards)
  - signposting (to specific patient groups, training, social services etc) – see Chapters 4, 5 and 6 for more ideas about practice systems that support self care as well as how individual practitioners do it
- the appropriateness of self care support provided – the extent to which self care services are geared to meeting patient needs. Involve patients or the practice patient forum in feeding back on this
- accessibility of self care support services – where located, opening times
- information about self care – type, options for non-English speakers
- publicity – the extent to which the public are aware of the type and availability of self care support provided
- skill mix – staffing levels
- training of staff – working within their competencies, sufficient opportunities for continuing professional development
- good communication with staff at all levels about promoting and supporting self care.

Once the audit has been undertaken and actions taken to address your findings, review your audit cycle to conclude whether:

- any underlying reasons for any failure to meet standards in relation to supporting self care were identified
- everyone participated in the actual audit measuring their performance
- everyone supported and adhered to any changes made as a result of audit

- proposed changes were implemented
- training needs that were identified were addressed
- any further audits were indicated, and if so whether they were undertaken
- the quality of patient care improved
- acceptable outcomes were used to measure any interventions or changes to patient care.

What to do

Design your audit of an aspect of how you and others in the practice are promoting and supporting self care around the steps of the audit cycle represented in Figure T9.1.

- Prioritise and select the topic of your audit, working with others in your team or practice.
- Set objectives: relating to the reason(s) why the audit is being carried out.
- Review the literature for that topic and agree the criteria and standards that you think are reasonable – look back at Chapter 2 for information as to how others have promoted and supported self care.
- Design the way in which you will do the audit.
- Collect the data and look at it.
- Feed back the findings; meet with colleagues or your team to discuss the findings and determine the reasons for the results.
- Make a timetabled action plan to implement any changes that are needed.
- Review your standards – should you keep the standards you previously set, are they unrealistic or not challenging enough?
- Re-audit – creating successive audit cycles.

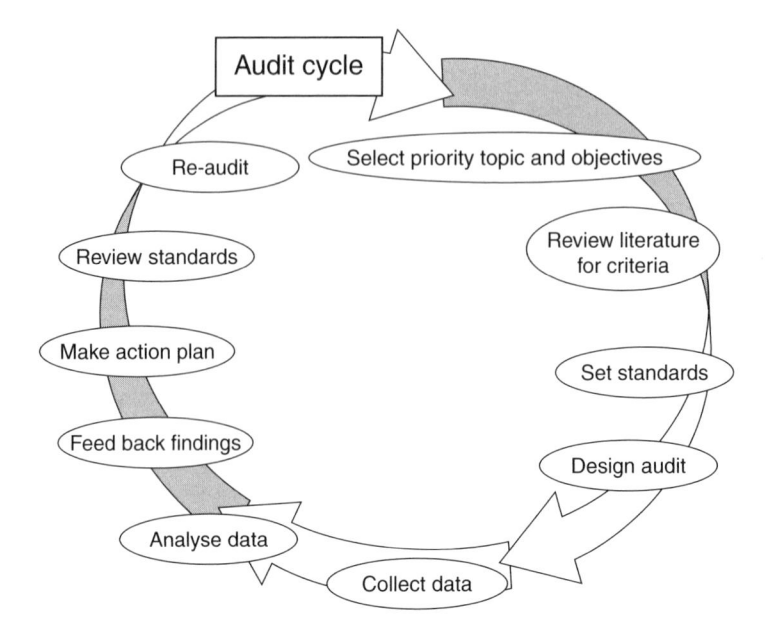

Figure T9.1: Steps in the audit cycle.

How it works (insight)

The audit will be worthwhile if the objectives of your audit are about:

- assessing whether or not standards are being met – in relation to promoting and supporting self care
- determining if standards are improving
- monitoring levels of compliance or concordance with treatment or self care advice and support
- changing inadequate current practice.

Whom to engage

Include those members of the PCT/practice team who are directly involved in the task being audited and those who will be collecting the data. Engage with patients to give you their perspective. Decide who is writing the audit protocol and who will search for evidence to enable you to set standards and criteria. Include in the team those who need to agree solutions or find resources if the audit shows that change is necessary. Appoint a lead if there is no-one in this role already. Link to others relevant to the audit who work in different settings: the local hospital, PCT, community clinic, social services, etc.

How much time you should allow

This will depend on the complexity of the audit, how much data gathering is involved etc.

What a facilitator should do

Ensure that the purpose and plan for the audit is clear, and that it concerns an important problem or issue.

What to do next

Follow the stages of the audit cycle, including re-audit after changes have been made.

What makes it work better

Being clear about the reason(s) for doing the audit, and that the objectives are linked to that. The objectives should be relevant and understandable to everyone taking part. The end results should be making improvements to patient care. The quality and nature of the end points of your audit should relate to the objective(s) you set for the audit. You need to have some idea of your end point(s) when you set the objective(s).

What can go wrong

The audit can be too complicated or resource intensive so that it founders halfway through. There may be no change possible once the initial stages of the audit have been completed and the problem is well described – which is demoralising for everyone concerned.

Tool 10

Training needs analysis

Why you should use this

Identifying training needs is a generic task that every practice team should be able to do.

When to use this

It is useful for a team leader, supervisor or manager when putting together the annual training plan for a team. Undertake this exercise at least annually as a routine, for everyone in the PCT or practice, or in a focused way when a new initiative or way of working is contemplated.

What to do

Compose an annual training plan for the PCT/practice team. Record information about staff training needs in respect of the essential or special services you provide (see Table T10.1).

Table T10.1: Training plan

Department or team: **Date:**

Healthcare area	Healthcare area 1	Healthcare area 2	Healthcare area 3
Service change required			
Expected benefit to patients			
People involved			
Training required			

How it works (insight)
Collecting information from various perspectives enables you to record current perceived training needs, and anticipate the new knowledge and skills and attitudes that will be required, for example, in developing an integrated resource to support self care. It is a good repository for the learning needs identified at people's appraisals from across your PCT/practice.

Whom to engage
Individuals and team leaders who represent a good cross-section of the workforce in your PCT/practice.

How much time you should allow
You will be lucky to complete this over a month's period, cajoling everyone to contribute information from appraisals and training needs questionnaires. The time to collate the responses and chase non-respondents will depend on the size of your organisation.

What a facilitator should do
Establish a routine so everyone in your PCT/practice contributes information about training needs at a particular time of year and can time annual appraisals accordingly. Agree a standard questionnaire to ascertain training needs so people know what to expect and can gather information proactively.

What to do next
Agree the format and timing of any training in relation to supporting self care, with team leaders and others who are key to providing information. Team leaders and line managers should agree what training an individual will undertake as a result.

What makes it work better
- Keeping any enquiry about training needs to a simple format, making it obvious that there will be resources to provide training to address needs.
- Collecting objective evidence of training needs.

What can go wrong
- Team leaders and others do not co-operate with completing the training needs enquiry, making analysis difficult.
- The process lags on over too long a time interval, or there is limited or inappropriate training on offer, and everyone regards the training needs analysis as a waste of time.

Tool 11

How well is your team functioning?

Why you should use this
Good teamwork does not just happen. Take time out as a team away from the workplace to review how you are working together.

When to use this
A team away day when the team is reviewing progress or preparing to promote a new initiative such as supporting self care.

What to do
Ask everyone to complete the quiz below.[1]

There is good communication between colleagues at work	usually/seldom/not at all
There is good communication between managers and staff	usually/seldom/not at all
Team members' functions are clear	usually/seldom/not at all
Staff are proud to be working in your practice/unit	usually/seldom/not at all
Doctors/managers resolve staff problems	usually/seldom/not at all
Staff are treated with respect by doctors and managers	usually/seldom/not at all
There is a person-friendly culture at work	usually/seldom/not at all
There are opportunities for staff for self-improvement	usually/seldom/not at all
Positive feedback about performance is the norm at work	usually/seldom/not at all
Staff are well trained for the tasks they are asked to do	usually/seldom/not at all
Team members' responsibilities are clear	usually/seldom/not at all
There is good leadership of the team	usually/seldom/not at all

Score: usually = 3, seldom = 1, not at all = 0.

Scores between 27 and 36: you have a well functioning team
Scores between 24 and 15: look at your weak areas and make plans for improvements
Scores of 15 and below: as you have a long way to go, it may be best for you to consider using an external consultant to help facilitate team development

How it works (insight)
Everyone should have an equal chance of giving their perspective as to how the team is functioning. Completing the quiz independently allows everyone to be honest.

Whom to engage
Everyone in the team.

How much time you should allow

Ten minutes to complete the quiz and whatever time it takes to collate the results. Then up to one hour to discuss the collated responses and what changes should be made to improve teamwork and relationships.

What a facilitator should do

Arrange for everyone to complete a copy of the quiz, anonymously. Collate the responses. Feed back the overall response to the team and facilitate the subsequent discussion about the way forward.

What to do next

Keep a watchful eye on the agreed changes being implemented and arrange a review with key members of the team of the progress made.

What makes it work better

Creation of the feeling and belief that every team member is valued.

What can go wrong

Team leaders can be affronted by feedback from others that reveals the team is not working as well as they believed. Team leaders may lack insight and refuse to take action despite constructive feedback and discussion from others in the team.

Reference

1. Chambers R and Davies M. *What Stress in Primary Care!* London: Royal College of General Practitioners; 1999.

Tool 12

Significant event audit

Why you should use this

Significant event auditing is a structured approach to reviewing events that have occurred in your PCT or practice.

When to use this

Choose an area relevant to your work, such as an unexpected adverse clinical event when a patient delayed seeking help from a GP or nurse as they were self caring for too long.

What to do

Discuss the completed significant event audit at a meeting of the GPs and nurses or local pharmacist, the primary care team or within a special interest group. Determine what lessons can be learnt, what areas require further work, how care can be improved, who is responsible for the action plan and by when.

Record significant events where someone experienced an adverse event or had a near miss.

1. Describe the incident.
2. Recount the effect on all of the participants.
3. Deduce the reasons for the event arising, through discussion, review of records, procedures etc.
4. Decide how you or others might have behaved differently and describe your options for how procedures might be changed to reduce or prevent recurrences.
5. Agree any changes that are needed, how they will be implemented, who will be responsible for what and when.
6. Re-audit later to see if the changes have worked. Give feedback to the team and acknowledge good care.

How it works (insight)

Significant event audits can give an understanding of the care that individual practitioners or the practice team deliver. While all significant events have the capacity to be identified as areas for improvement, they can also demonstrate good or appropriate care. Adverse events are where something clearly has gone wrong, and the team needs to establish what happened, what was preventable and how to respond. Adverse events might include a patient's complaint, an allergic reaction to a drug bought over-the-counter as a form of self care, or a prescribing error that came about as home remedies clashed with the prescribed drug, for instance.

Whom to engage
Everyone involved in the factors leading up to the significant event, who was connected with the event when it happened, and who can contribute to the range of solutions to prevent it happening again.

How much time you should allow
At least an hour for initial discussion of the significant event. Then as much time as needed to gather information about the factors leading up to the event, considering possible changes, recruiting support for the action plan, and subsequent change and review of progress leading to re-audit.

What a facilitator should do
One person records the discussion and agreed actions as described above. Bring everyone together, chair the review of the event in non-confrontational manner, and see through all the stages of the significant event audit.

What to do next
Maintain progress in undertaking the activities in the action plan, then re-auditing.

What makes it work better
Most significant incidents do not have one cause. Usually there are faults in the system, which are compounded by someone, or several people, being careless, tired, overworked or ill-informed. Cultivate an atmosphere of openness and discussion without blame. Look for *all* the causes and try to remedy as many as possible to prevent the situation from arising again.

What can go wrong
An atmosphere of blame and recrimination will mean that people involved will hide the incident and no-one will be able to prevent it happening again.

Tool 13

PART/workload assessment

Why you should use this

To help you as a practice prioritise which conditions you will tackle next to provide self care support. To review the frequency with which patients are consulting for specific conditions in your practice or a group of practices if you are thinking of it from a PCT perspective.

When to use this

In a practice planning day or team meeting – working in a group.

What to do

Take some of the conditions listed in Box T13.1. These may be conditions for which patients might undertake more self care, or conditions where GPs and nurses are seeing patients who they believe do not need to consult them directly. Place these selected conditions in the matrix of Box T13.2 according to whether they frequently occur and, if they do, the workload implications for the GP or (triage) nurse. Either estimate the frequency and complexity of such consultations as a team, or collect or collate baseline data first.

1 Take only the conditions you placed in the high demand/low complexity sector (bottom left quadrant of Box T13.2) and place each one in as many quadrants as you wish in Box T13.3.
2 Prevention, awaiting resolution, relief and tolerance of symptoms for a particular condition may all be relevant self care options to guide a patient to or train them for; if so, write that specific condition in each of the four sectors of Box T13.3. You might start with the three (or more) health conditions for which there is highest demand and least complexity.
3 Take each of the conditions you placed in the matrix in Box T13.3 and place them in a copy of Table T13.1 indicating which members of the practice team are best placed to provide prevention, await resolution, relieve symptoms or encourage tolerance. Add extra rows to Table T13.1 to accommodate other health professionals or patients/carers if they are part of your team too.

How it works (insight)

It allows a practice team to prioritise one or more conditions for which there is potential opportunity to minimise practice team workload, with similar or improved patient health and wellbeing outcomes. Thinking of the four components of self care support brings a wide perspective.

Whom to engage

The exercise is suitable for everyone in the practice team with contact with patients, or who has a role to promote or support self care. Include local community pharmacists and interested staff from the PCT to gain a wider perspective and collaboration.

How much time you should allow

As long as someone has collected baseline data on workload for identified conditions, up to an hour with ensuing discussion. Longer for subsequent action planning.

What a facilitator should do

Urge individual practice team members to subsequent action to promote and support self care as part of a co-ordinated plan.

What to do next

Arrange a review meeting for the first conditions prioritised for report on progress, barriers to action, patients' responses. If all is going well, include other conditions; if progress is slow, focus on solutions that will re-affirm the culture of promoting and supporting self care.

What makes it work better

Everyone involved should understand the potential benefits to practice workload and patients' wellbeing when patients undertake more self care. You could use the same template as Table T13.1 for team members to record what they are already doing for that condition prior to the team meeting or discussion, to get individual staff thinking what self care support is already being provided that can be built upon.

What can go wrong

Practice team members may find it difficult to relinquish 'professional power' to patients and encourage them to self care. If the self care support is not provided with patient safety as core, there may be risks to patients' wellbeing if the self care they adopt is not appropriate or in line with conventional health care.

Box T13.1: Examples of conditions for which patients consult a GP or practice team – that might be amenable to elements of supported self care as a starter

Acne	Impotence
Acute constipation	Irritable bowel syndrome
Acute diarrhoea	Knee disorder
Allergic/acute rhinitis/hayfever	Menopause
Allergy	Menstruation disorder
Anxiety	Migraine
Asthma	Mouth ulcer
Backache	Nappy rash
Breathlessness/wheezing	Nausea
Chronic constipation	Obesity
Conjunctivitis	Oral thrush
Cough	Pain in neck
Cystitis	Palpitations
Depression	Premenstrual tension
Diabetes – type 1	Psoriasis
Diabetes – type 2	Rash
Dizziness/giddiness/faintness	Sciatica
Dry skin	Sinusitis
Dyspepsia/indigestion/heartburn	Smoking cessation
Dysuria	Sore throat
Eczema	Stress
Fever/pyrexia	Tiredness
Frozen shoulder/pain	Tonsillitis
Gastroenteritis	Upper respiratory tract infection
Haemorrhoids	Urinary incontinence
Head lice	Vaginal discharge
Hypertension	Varicose veins
Ingrowing nail	Verucca/wart
Insomnia/sleep disturbances	Vomiting

Box T13.2: GP/practice team workload associated with condition

Frequency consultations occur

	High	Low
High Workload on GP/practice team (complexity and/or length of consultation) Low		

Box T13.3: Conditions to prioritise for self care support

Prevention	Await resolution
Relieve symptoms	Tolerance

Table T13.1: Checklist of practice team members' roles in supporting self care for each selected condition

Role	Prevention	Await resolution	Relieve symptoms	Tolerance
GP				
Nurse				
Practice manager				
Health care assistant				
Receptionist				
Pharmacist				
Other				

Tool 14

Moving through change

Why you should use this
People tend to resist change, especially when they work in a busy NHS setting. By understanding the current difficulties and the new vision, people will be pulled towards a change.

When to use this
When you are planning to make a change such as promoting a self care culture in your PCT or practice.

What to do
Look at the equation below. Work through what you can do about the four factors on the left hand side of the equation:

$$\text{Dissatisfaction} \times \text{Vision} \times \text{Capacity} \times \text{First steps} \rightarrow \text{Lower resistance}$$

Factor 1: dissatisfaction
- How satisfied is the person/the people who will be affected by the change, with the current state of things?
- Is any dissatisfaction shared with their colleagues?
- How is the dissatisfaction understood and experienced?

Factor 2: vision
- What do they want for their patients, themselves and their colleagues?
- What are their values and beliefs, goals and desires?
- What could the new system look like?

Factor 3: capacity
- What resources are needed to achieve the change?
- How can resources be generated or shared?
- Have people shown in the past that they are willing to try out new ideas?
- Is there anyone who has demonstrated the energy and capability to make changes?

Factor 4: first steps
- What first steps could people undertake which everyone agrees would be moving in the right direction?

How it works (insight)
Generally, it is better to pull people towards a change rather than push people into it. Realise that the costs and risks of maintaining the status quo may outweigh the risks and uncertainty of making the change.

Whom to engage
Any individual or team involved in planning for and making change happen.

How much time you should allow
An hour initially, with ongoing review in the course of the change process.

What a facilitator should do
Facilitate the initial discussion, and keep tabs on progress at and between the intermittent reviews while the change is underway.

What to do next
Organise review meetings as the change gets underway, looking for positive drivers to keep up the momentum for change.

What makes it work better
Find role models to enthuse people affected by change.

What can go wrong
Change is so dramatic and sudden that there is insufficient time or positive momentum to create the climate for change to happen naturally.

Tool 15

Keep a reflective learning log

Why you should do this
You should have a permanent record of your learning to keep in your portfolio. Then you have evidence of your learning activities if required for supervision, appraisal or accreditation. It will help you reflect on your experiences at work and apply what you have learnt more effectively.

When to use this
You could use this technique over the first three or six months that you actively promote and support patients' self care. Then discuss or review what you have written with a mentor, manager or tutor or supervisor.

What to do
Pick out the most personally significant experiences on a particular day and record what you learnt from the experience. This will involve you reflecting on:

- what was most significant
- why this was personally significant
- what you learnt
- any actions you propose to take as a result.

Use the log to record other thoughts, ideas, insights and feelings. You might also include what worked for you and what did not, and the reasons for that.

How it works (insight)
It helps you to reflect on the significance of what and how you are learning.

How much time you should allow
Set aside time to complete the logbook at the end of a day or an event.

What to do next
Look at your learning style and whether other ways of learning and working might suit you better.

What makes it work better
- Practise reflecting about your learning and work.
- Being self-motivated.

What can go wrong
- Reluctant learners do not want to spend time reflecting on their learning.
- People who do not prioritise time for reflection.

Tool 16

Reduce time pressures at work

Why you should use this
To plan to stay in control of your workload.

When to use this
In a workshop or as homework.

What to do
Look at the suggestions in Table T16.1 for reducing time pressures, from the perspectives of an individual and a PCT or practice. Add any other ideas to both lists. Work in pairs to make action plans for up to five specific ways of reducing time pressures in your work setting – what you can do yourself and what your PCT or practice can do (Table T16.2).

How it works (insight)
This forces you to realise the varied options that there are for reducing time pressures and that you are not helpless. It also helps you to understand that you cannot reduce time pressures as an individual, in isolation from the rest of your organisation.

Whom to engage
Managers and staff – anyone and everyone.

Table T16.1: Suggestions for reducing time pressures

What you can do as an individual	*What the PCT or practice can do*
Plan well in advance to avoid crises	Plan well in advance to avoid crises
Allow 10% of your time for unexpected tasks	Organise time management training for staff
Do not book a meeting too close to a previous commitment which may overrun	Match staff numbers to volume of work
Build in time for reflection and planning	Organise realistic work plans
Minimise interruptions	Discourage social chit chat in work time
Make maximum use of technology	Make maximum use of technology
Other:	Other:

Table T16.2: Action points to reduce time pressures, and what you will do:

	As an individual	And when	As an organisation	And when
1				
2				
3				
4				

How much time you should allow
Encourage brainstorming and discussion by allowing about 90 minutes for the exercise.

What a facilitator should do
Have plenty of illustrative examples that have worked elsewhere when people have tackled time pressures. Intervene if participants get distracted by talking about negative effects of time pressures rather than making positive plans.

What to do next
Try to arrange a follow-up review of intended actions – maybe as pairs of participants or a working party at organisational level.

What makes it work better
- A mixed group of staff from different disciplines, managers and clinicians will bring individual and organisational perspectives and hopefully improve the subsequent action plans.
- An external person or new member of staff might feed in their relatively independent views of what time pressures they perceive and the effort put into reducing such pressures.

What can go wrong
It is all very well making resolutions – quite another to put those resolutions into practice.

Tool 17

Check out whether self care support is a priority for training and whether the way in which you plan to learn about it is appropriate

Why you should use this
If promoting and supporting self care is a new priority for you and/or your PCT or practice, you will need to update your personal development plan and the PCT/practice business plan.

When to use this
When you are checking out the extent to which promoting and supporting self care is a priority for the PCT or practice you work in; and your current knowledge and skills, to deduce what resources for development you need for your future role.

What to do
Interested individuals should complete the self-assessment on pp. 218–20.

How it works (insight)
It is a structured way to evaluate the extent to which knowledge and skills are required for a new role, and to weight their importance against other learning and service development needs.

Whom to engage
The self-assessment form should be useful for any member of staff where changes are happening such that their role will be affected.

How much time you should allow
Fifteen minutes upwards depending on the degree to which homework is required to collect information about PCT/practice policies and plans, to score current knowledge and skills, or to discuss perception of what is required with a mentor, supervisor or line manager.

What a facilitator should do

Take time to encourage individuals to complete the self-assessment form and discuss their identified learning needs with their line manager or other, and plan/pursue learning activities.

What to do next

Work with educational lead or trainer in the PCT/practice to distribute the self-assessment learning needs form in organised way. Encourage someone to collate completed forms and plan learning events to meet needs. Link into the personal development planning/appraisal process of the PCT or practice.

What makes it work better

Plenty of resources to meet learning and service development needs!

What can go wrong

Individuals completing the forms according to their 'wants' rather than their PCT's or practice's service needs.

Self-assessment: promoting and supporting self care for patients

1 How have you identified your learning need(s) in relation to self care?

    PCT requirement ☐
    Practice business plan ☐
    Clinical governance: patient safety requirement ☐
    Job requirement ☐
    Appraisal need ☐
    New to post ☐
    Individual decision ☐
    Patient feedback ☐
    Other ☐

2 Have you discussed or planned your learning needs with anyone else?

    Yes ☐
    No ☐

    If yes, who? ....

3 What are the learning need(s) and/or objective(s) in terms of:

- *Knowledge*: what new information do you hope to gain to help you do this?

....

- *Skills*: what should you be able to do differently as a result of undertaking this development?

  ....

- *Behaviour/professional practice*: how will this impact on the way you do things?

  ....

4 Details and date of desired development activity:

   ....

5 Details of any previous training and/or experience you have in relation to supporting self care:

   ....

6 Your current performance in this area against the requirements of your job:

   Need significant development in this area ☐
   Need some development in this area ☐
   Satisfactory in this area ☐
   Do well in this area ☐

7 Level of job relevance that supporting self care has to your role and responsibilities:

   Has no relevance to job ☐
   Has some relevance ☐
   Relevant to job ☐
   Very relevant ☐
   Essential to job ☐

8 Describe what aspect of your job and how the proposed education/training is relevant:

   ....

9 Is additional support needed in identifying a suitable development activity?

   Yes ☐
   No ☐
   What do you need?

   ....

10 Describe the differences or improvements for you, your practice or your PCT as a result of undertaking this activity?

   ....

11 Determine the priority of your proposed educational/training activity:

   Urgent ☐
   High ☐
   Medium ☐
   Low ☐

12 Describe how the proposed activity will meet your learning needs rather than any other type of course or training on the topic:

   ....

13 If you had a free choice would you want to learn this?   Yes/No

   If *not*, why not? (please circle all that apply):
   waste of time
   already done it
   not relevant to my work, career goals
   other

   If *yes*, what reasons are most important to you (put in rank order):
   improve my performance
   increase my knowledge
   get promotion
   just interested
   be better than my colleagues
   do a more interesting job
   be more confident
   it will help me
   it will help patients and/or members of the public

Tool 18

Draw up a personal map of support mechanisms in your life

Why you should do this
To realise the components of your life that lend you support, that you can build upon to promote your own self care. Or use the exercise with a patient to enable them to adopt a self care approach.

When to use this
With a group of people who have been meeting regularly and feel comfortable sharing feelings. Alternatively you can use it yourself as an individual with or without a facilitator or mentor.

What to do
- *Stage 1*: draw yourself in the middle of a piece of plain paper. Then draw pictures to represent all the sources of support in your life – people, things, situations, environment etc. Link each picture to you in the centre with a line (*see* the example following).
- *Stage 2*: add in drawings of what other sources of support you have used in the past but not employed for a while, and add other pictures of what extra sources of support you would like to have. Link each picture to you in the centre of the page.
- *Stage 3*: draw in the barriers that stop you using these sources of support across the line linking that particular source with you.
- *Stage 4*: share your personal support map with someone else. Discuss which are your strongest sources of support, which ones you would like to enhance, the presence of the barriers that stop you making more of your sources of support, and what is missing.

How it works (insight)
It helps you to acknowledge and review the extent and type of the sources of support that exist at work or outside work. It may give you insight into how sources of support have withered away, or how you are taking some sources for granted and not devoting enough quality time to your supporters. You might recognise the barriers that stop you from spending time and effort on leisure activities or maintaining relationships.

Whom to engage
The exercise works for anyone who wants to review and maintain or build up support mechanisms.

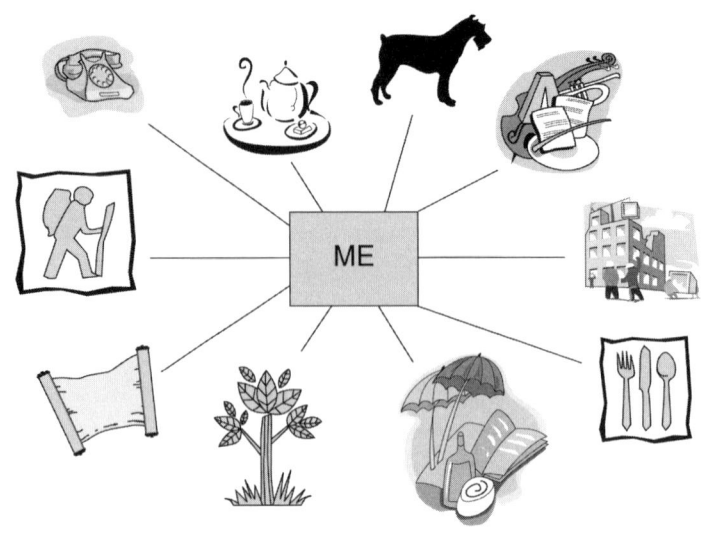

Personal support mapping exercise

Figure T18.1: Example of a personal support map (reproduced from Chambers *et al.*).[1]

How much time you should allow

Twenty to 30 minutes for Stages 1, 2 and 3, with another 20 minutes for Stage 4.

What a facilitator should do

Keep the exercise moving. Discourage people from intense or emotional discussion at Stage 4 if the exercise is being undertaken in a group setting as a preliminary activity to other educational activities.

What to do next

Encourage participants to make a plan to remove at least one barrier, to enhance at least one source of support.

What makes it work better

An atmosphere of trust and mutual respect between participants.

What can go wrong

One or more individuals may become distressed if they suddenly realise the lack of sources of support in their lives.

An example of a personal support map is shown in Figure T18.1.

Reference

1 Chambers R, Schwartz A and Boath E. *Beating Stress in the NHS*. Oxford: Radcliffe Medical Press; 2003.

Tool 19

Assess your consultation skills and style

Why you should use this
To help you to analyse your approach and achievements in patient consultations.

When to use this
Tate describes five tasks to be covered by a health professional in a consultation with a patient.[1] We've added a sixth to focus on supporting self care.

What to do
Use the checklist in Table T19.1 to review the extent to which you complete the six tasks for individual patients. Start with 10 patients picked at random from several surgeries or clinics (e.g. one or two per surgery or clinic) and complete the checklist after each session while the consultation is still fresh in your mind. Or review a series of consecutive consultations (e.g. the first or last five patients from two surgeries or clinics).

How it works (insight)
It should help you to consider the extent to which you keep your determination to support self care, in balance with the reasons that the patient is consulting with you.

Whom to engage
Any health professional can do this.

How much time you should allow
The minimum time this exercise should take is 60 minutes, allowing a little time for reflection.

What a facilitator should do
Sell the importance of supporting self care as an integral part of a consultation, rather than the dominating feature.

What to do next
Debrief with a colleague or as a team, and reflect on whether your support for self care is appropriately introduced in most of your consultations.

Table T19.1: Check out how comprehensive your approach is in patient consultations and if they include support for self care

Component of consultation	Whether you did this (tick if so)
1 Discover the reason(s) your patient has come to see you	
elicit the patient's account of the symptom(s) that made him or her turn to you	
obtain relevant information about the patient's social and occupational circumstances	
explore your patient's health understanding	
enquire about other problems	
2 Define clinical problems	
obtain additional information about critical symptoms and details of the patient's medical history	
assess your patient's condition by examination if appropriate	
make a working diagnosis	
3 Address your patient's problem(s)	
assess the severity of the presenting problem	
together with the patient, choose an appropriate form of management	
involve your patient in their self care plan to an appropriate extent	
try to achieve a shared care plan	
4 Explain the problem(s) to your patient	
tailor the explanation to the needs of your patient	
ensure that the explanation is understood and accepted by your patient	
try to achieve a shared understanding of the problem(s)	
5 Make effective use of the consultation	
make efficient use of resources	
establish and maintain an effective relationship with your patient	
give opportunistic health advice where appropriate	
6 Support self care	
discuss future prevention of the condition or health problem	
explain how to wait for resolution of the current or future health problem	
explain how self care can alleviate health condition	
encourage tolerance of the health condition – as appropriate	

What makes it work better

Someone could video or audiotape their consultations and ask a colleague to complete the checklists above, then compare their own and their colleagues' responses. The patients concerned might complete the checklist, then the health professional compare their own and the patient's assessments and consider if they are matched, and if not, why not.

What can go wrong

An individual health professional without insight completes the checklists which then serve to reinforce their pattern of consulting behaviour.

Reference

1 Tate P. *The Doctor's Communication Handbook*. Oxford: Radcliffe Medical Press; 2001.

Tool 20

Determine your consulting style

Why you should use this
An aspect that you could look at in respect of assessing your consultation skills is to determine your consulting style, and the extent to which you are health professional- or patient-centred.

When to use this
As a health professional who is reviewing the extent to which their normal approach is to be patient-centred and enable patients to receive the care that they seek.

What to do
Rate where you think you usually are on the scale in Box T20.1. You can increase the objectivity of this exercise by asking others to complete it about you. You could ask colleagues to complete the scale judging by their experience of sharing patients with you.

How it works (insight)
Doing this exercise should help you to consider the extent to which you are patient-centred or health professional-centred, to keep your determination to promote and support self care, in balance with the reasons that the patient is consulting with you.

Whom to engage
Any health professional in the practice can do this.

How much time you should allow
The minimum time this exercise should take is 50 minutes, allowing a little time for reflection and involving ten patients in giving you feedback.

What the facilitator should do
Encourage health professionals you are facilitating, to support self care in a way that is individualised to the patients who are consulting.

Determine your consulting style

Box T20.1: What sort of consulter are you? Are you health professional- or patient-centred?

I do most of the talking	5	4	3	2	1	2 3 4 5	The patient does most of the talking
I ask mostly closed questions	5	4	3	2	1	2 3 4 5	I ask mostly open questions
I am mainly interested in problems	5	4	3	2	1	2 3 4 5	I am mainly interested in people
It is my medical agenda that is most important	5	4	3	2	1	2 3 4 5	It is the patient's agenda that is most important
I feel responsible for my patient's problems	5	4	3	2	1	2 3 4 5	The patient is responsible for their own problems
I usually try to maintain, control and guide the consultation	5	4	3	2	1	2 3 4 5	I usually let my patient control and guide the consultation
I usually choose care options and plans	5	4	3	2	1	2 3 4 5	The patient usually chooses management options and plans
I believe in explaining	5	4	3	2	1	2 3 4 5	I believe in reaching a shared understanding

In relation to the above criteria, where are you usually on the scale below?

A health professional-centred consulter	5	4	3	2	1	2 3 4 5	A patient-centred consulter

(Box T20.1 is reproduced from Tate P. *The Doctor's Communication Handbook*. Oxford: Radcliffe Medical Press; 2001, with permission.)

What to do next
Sell the importance of supporting self care as an integral part of a patient-centred consultation.

What makes it work better
It will be better if you ask up to ten patients to complete the scale from their perspectives – and compare whether they agree with your own rating if you dare!

What can go wrong
- An individual health professional without insight completes the chart for a variety of patients, rating themselves incorrectly as being patient-centred, which then serves to reinforce their pattern of consulting behaviour.
- Health professionals who do not care whether they are rated as being health professional- or patient-centred so long as they get through their everyday work.

Tool 21

Self care aware consultation style: encouraging, guiding and providing support to patients to adopt self care

Why you should use this

Practise supporting patients to adopt self care as an integral part of their consultations, if you do not do so already, using this tool to reflect on how and when you can include self care support in your everyday practice.

When to use this

When you are upskilling your approach to supporting self care – initially or to review your progress.

What to do

Read through the sequence of boxes that follow on pp. 232–3, to realise what good practice you are aiming at in your self care aware consultations. You could complete Table T21.1 as part of a training session during role play, where you are the health professional whom a fictitious patient is consulting. Then others observing the role play or playing the part of patient can comment on your behaviour. Alternatively you could audiotape or video maybe three consultations after which you review the extent to which you adopted any or all of the eight types of behaviour described below in the table. Then make conclusions, resolve to improve your practice, and review at a later date.

Examples of fictitious scenarios are: 'The fictitious patient has had a bad back for the past 10 days', or 'The fictitious patient consults the GP to ask for tablets to help her to lose weight'.

How it works (insight)

It gives you the opportunity to reflect on the extent to which you are using the consultation to encourage and support self care, in an optimal way that is challenging and motivating for the patient.

Whom to engage

Any health professional who wants to improve their skills in supporting self care to individual patients.

Table T21.1: Recording your behaviour

Behaviour	Your comments
Challenging:	
question the person's assumptions about their health and wellbeing. Encourage the person to think things through.	
offer experience of other patients' changes (e.g. use anonymised patient stories): draw parallels with others' experiences 'When they faced a similar situation, they . . .'	
Guiding:	
suggest where to look for new knowledge or insights. Point the person in the right direction	
Suggesting:	
'why don't you try this?'	
'you may find this will help'	
'look at . . .'	
Encouraging:	
help the person to reflect on previous achievements	
motivate about new goals. Build on confidence	
Stimulating:	
direct the person's enthusiasm to where it will have the greatest impact	
Body language:	
interested posture, good eye contact, being open	
Environmental factors:	
comfortable setting, not across a desk; protected from interruptions; with an agreed allocation time	

How much time you should allow

Allow 45 minutes for discussion of a role play of one consultation lasting 10–15 minutes. Allow 1.5 to 2 hours to review and reflect on a series of say three audio- or videotaped consultations.

What a facilitator should do

Set up the exercise so that those involved feel comfortable, use constructive feedback, give the observers and then those in role play a chance to feed back on what has gone well and what might be improved. Sum up and make conclusions about necessary changes to practice and behaviour.

What to do next

Repeat the exercise and review a series of consultations, say three months later, to check out how things are going and if patients are more likely to adopt self care. Follow up specific patients to monitor their progress – e.g. they make less frequent consultations with the GP or practice nurse about trivial symptoms or minor ailments.

What makes it work better

Welcome the objective feedback of others. Involve a colleague in critiquing your consultations so that you can compare your review of the types of behaviour you're using with their assessment of you.

What can go wrong

Your initial enthusiasm might founder under the pressure of other commitments without protected study and reflection time.

Recommended sequence for a self care aware consultation exercise

---

1 What is a 'self care aware consultation'?

It involves:

- all contacts with the wide primary care team members
- using the person's own potential for independent action
- building a set of skills and attitudes for future use
- providing support where necessary.

---

2 What is a 'self care aware consultation'?

The outcome is:

- a coherence across the primary care team
- patients and carers building on their existing skills
- more patient-centred consultations in general practice.

---

3 The keys to a 'self care aware consultation'

- Understanding the patient's self care journey.
- Supporting the patient's self care decisions.

---

4 Types of 'self care aware consultations'

- *One example*: self care for self-limiting illness.
- *Other examples*: long term conditions, support for carers, lifestyle choices, risk awareness.

---

5 Understanding the patient's self care journey

- Taking a history that includes self care
  - for how long have the symptom/s been present?
  - what has the patient already tried? Hot water bottle, resting, taking OTC medicines, complementary products or food supplements, seeing an allied health professional or alternative practitioner?
  - and for how long?

6 Understanding the patient's self care journey

- What have you already tried?
- How long have you tried this?
- What were you trying to achieve by doing/taking this?
- Has it worked and how?
- Have you stopped doing what you tried – and why?
- What could you do next time?

7 Understanding the patient's self care journey

Answers will reveal:

- how willing the patient is to think about their health options
- the potential for change now and in the future
- the patient's reasons for consulting
- the possibility of coming back to advise on self care at the end of the consultation.

8 Supporting the patient's self care decisions

- Endorse current self care practice and encourage it for the future.
- Ensure understanding of the right time period for self care before the need for professional help is to be sought.
- Endorse consultation with other professionals in the primary care team.
- Use written information where possible to support advice and enforcement of self care.

9 Aide mémoire

- What have you already tried?
- How long have you tried this?
- What were you trying to achieve by doing/taking this?
- Has it worked and how?
- Have you stopped doing what you tried – and why?
- What could you do next time?

Appendix 1

Useful resources

BestTreatments: www.besttreatments.co.uk
  Helps patients make informed choices about treatments, based on the best available research published in *Clinical Evidence*

Department of Health: www.dh.gov.uk/SelfCare
  Provides guidance on how to support self care; with a wealth of evidence on the effectiveness and cost effectiveness of self care support

Developing Patient Partnerships (DPP): www.dpp.org.uk
  The DPP specialises in producing health education campaigns to encourage better communication between the public and health professionals, helping people take control of their health and access NHS service effectively

Diabetes Education and Self Management for Ongoing and Newly Diagnosed (DESMOND): www.cgsupport.nhs.uk and www.desmond-project.org.uk
  Aimed at people with diabetes but also useful for health professionals

DIPEx (Database of Individual Patient Experiences): www.dipex.org
  Audio and video interviews with people describing their personal experiences of various medical problems

DISCERN: www.discern.org.uk
  Brief questionnaire that allows users to assess the quality of information on treatment choices for health problems

Dose Adjustment For Normal Eating (DAFNE): www.dafne.uk.com

Expert Patients Programme: www.expertpatients.nhs.uk
  Provides self care skills training to people with long term conditions

Family Doctor Books: www.familydoctor.co.uk
  A resource for doctors and pharmacists to recommend to patients

Lab Tests Online UK: http://labtestsonline.org.uk
  Provides information for patients and caregivers, relating to clinical laboratory tests that are part of routine care, or used in the diagnosis or treatment of a broad range of conditions and diseases

Medicines Partnership: www.concordance.org and www.medicines-partnership.org
  Aims to put principles of concordance into practice

MEDLINEplus: http://medlineplus.gov
  Provides authoritative health information from the US National Library of Medicine on over 600 diseases and conditions

National Library for Health: www.library.nhs.uk
  A co-ordinated network of NHS library services and resources. Provides links and guidance and guidelines, evidence-based and clinical databases, journals, books plus the contents of the National electronic Library for Health – most resources are freely available

NHS Direct Interactive: available on Sky but soon to be available through Freeview
  Digital TV service providing information on health, self care and NHS services

NHS Direct Online: www.nhsdirect.nhs.uk
    The NHS Direct Online service mirrors the NHS Direct phone service, providing information online for patients and the public. It includes health news, information on healthy living and common health problems, a guide to NHS services and information on conditions and treatments

Patient Voices: www.patientvoices.org.uk
    Patient Voices are 'digital stories' produced by Pilgrim Projects, that use video, audio, text and music to convey patients' stories. They 'aim to touch the hearts of managers, clinicians and others striving to improve the quality of health care'

Proprietary Association of Great Britain (PAGB): www.pagb.org.uk

Working in Partnership Programme (WiPP): www.wipp.nhs.uk

Appendix 2

Record sheet to plan and describe your progress in supporting self care

Record your discussions, your action plan, your resource requirements and the outcomes that you expect – for your focus on self care of your chosen condition. Use the form below to record evidence that demonstrates you have achieved what you have planned.

Your prioritised topic for which you will provide self care support

Your team includes:

Team discussion

What you do next includes

What extra resources might this require?

Record sheet to plan and describe your progress

The outcomes might include:

How would you demonstrate that you have achieved your outcomes?

At a subsequent date record your actions completed and outcomes achieved

Actions:

1

2

3

Other:

Outcomes achieved (list them and label them in terms of the self care support approach as to whether it relates to **P**revention, **A**wait resolution, **R**elief of symptoms or **T**olerate symptoms):

Table A2.1: Role and responsibilities checklist

For each task tick the box for each team member who has a role or responsibility – then note your role and responsibilities for the task.

Completed by _____

Project team member

Task	Doctor	Practice nurse	Patient or carer	Reception team	Practice manager	Pharmacist	Pharmacy assistant	PCT	What are the roles and responsibilities?

INDEX

ABPI *see* Association of the British Pharmaceutical Industry
accident and emergency (A&E) 66, 85, 86, 107, 132
action learning sets 30, 31, 43, 45
action plans
    evaluation 119
    general practice teams 46, 49–51
    patient pathways 127, 138, 148, 151, 154, 157, 161
    PCTs 31, 32, 34, 38
    strategy and action plan (Tool 2) 32, 36, 46, 176–80
acupuncture 73, 74, 101, 103, 112, 143
Addison's disease 68
advanced services 81, 87, 89, 95
A&E *see* accident and emergency
Agenda for Change 69
AHPs *see* allied health professionals
alcohol 9, 103, 104
algorithms
    general practice teams 44, 45, 50
    long term conditions 23
    patient pathways 143, 161, 166
    PCTs 33
    pharmacy teams 81
    self care guides 21
allergies 104, 157, 165, 204
allied health professionals (AHPs) xi, 32, 45, 53
antibiotics
    cough and colds 159, 161, 162, 166–8
    educational interventions 18, 21
    self-limiting problems 84
    sore throat 126, 128, 129, 133, 134–5
anticoagulant therapy 23, 38, 99
antidepressants 76, 145
anxiety 25, 142
appraisal 36, 47, 69, 120–1, 201, 213, 218
arthritis 19, 20, 23, 74, 91, 104
aspirin 97, 152
assistive technologies 24
Association of the British Pharmaceutical Industry (ABPI) 107
asthma
    cough and colds 164, 165, 167

    educational interventions 21
    evaluation 118, 122
    long term conditions 22, 87–9
    overview of self care 7, 8
    PART model 16–17
    patient pathway
        case study 146–51
        self care 152–7
    patient's perspective 59–60, 104, 108
    pharmacy teams 87–9
audiotapes 18, 225, 229, 231
audit (Tool 9) *see also* significant event audit
    evaluation 122
    general practice teams 46, 51
    overview 197–9
    patient pathways 134, 164
    PCTs 35, 41
    pharmacy teams 83, 91, 93, 96–8
autonomy 9, 18, 59, 61, 157

The Back Book 138, 139, 143
back pain
    competence 72–4
    complementary medicine 112
    educational interventions 19
    evaluation 118
    minor ailment scheme 84, 138
    PART model 17, 142–3
    patient pathway
        case study 136–41
        self care 142–5
    pharmacy teams 84, 138
    work 110
barriers
    change 115, 116, 189
    general practice teams 46, 49, 50, 52
    PCTs 32, 40
    personal support mapping 221, 222
    support groups 108
Belbin, RM 47
benzodiazepines 145
BestTreatments 21, 68, 94, 234
beta blockers 152
Beth Johnson Foundation 20
Better Information, Better Choices, Better Health 6

blame 11, 114, 205
Blantyre/North Hamilton SIP 91
blood pressure
    educational interventions 19
    long term conditions 23, 87, 90
    overview of self care 10, 25
    patient's perspective 68, 102, 108, 109
    pharmacy teams 82, 87, 90, 91–4
body mass index (BMI) 87, 90, 92
Boots pharmacies 89, 92–3
British Medical Association 105
British Thoracic Society 148
bronchitis 167
Building on the Best 5
Burnley PCT 106–7

CAM *see* complementary and alternative medicine
cancer 94, 104, 144, 167
care plans 9, 154–7
carers 4, 48–9, 104, 109, 127, 130, 141
CBT *see* cognitive behavioural therapy
Centor scores 133, 134
change
    cycle of change 65
    force-field analysis 173
    general practice teams 50, 52
    moving through change (Tool 14) 40, 50, 211–12
    moving to self care culture 114–17
    PCTs 40
    PDSA 188, 189
    SWOT analysis 181
Chartered Society of Physiotherapy 104, 110
CHD *see* coronary heart disease
CHIC *see* Consumer Health Information Centre
children
    back pain 144
    cough and colds 159–61, 165–8
    educational interventions 18
    health and social services 9
    PART model 17
    patient's perspective 105
    sore throat 131, 132, 134
chiropractors 103, 111, 143
chloramphenicol 85, 97
cholesterol 87, 90

chronic obstructive pulmonary disease (COPD) 87, 148, 152, 167
Clinical Evidence 21, 143, 145, 234
clinical governance 31, 49, 96, 97
Cochrane Collaboration 111, 134, 168
codeine 137, 138, 144
cognitive behavioural therapy (CBT) 20, 59, 60, 145
colds
    asthma 89, 153
    educational interventions 18, 19
    minor ailment scheme 84, 138
    overview of self care 5, 7
    PART model 153, 166–7
    patient pathway
        case study 159–64
        self care 165–8
    sore throat 125, 131
communication
    audit 197
    health professionals 53, 54–6, 57, 69
    infrastructure and resource matrix 195
    overview of self care 6, 8
    PCTs 32
    risk and safety 11
    teams 47, 202
community pharmacists
    contract 81, 96, 98
    evaluation 121
    general practice teams 43, 45, 49
    long term conditions 86–9
    minor ailment scheme 84–6
    patient pathways 128, 130, 138, 141, 149, 162, 164
    prescription linked interventions 91, 92
    quality and audit 97, 98
    self-limiting problems 82, 83
    signposting 66
    teamwork 24, 81, 96, 99–100, 108
competence 53–4, 62, 69–74
complementary and alternative (CAM) medicine
    back pain 73, 74
    cough and colds 167
    health professionals 56, 73, 74, 76
    patient's perspective 56, 101, 102, 104, 111–12
    pharmacy teams 96
    promoting wellbeing 11
    risk and safety 76

Index

compliance 15, 17, 32, 61, 89, 97, 199
concordance 59, 61–2, 148, 150, 199
confidentiality 24, 57, 108, 128
conjunctivitis 84, 85, 138
Connexions 110, 111
conscious (in)competence 72
consultations
   consultation content scale 41, 51, 55, 223–5
   consulting style scale 41, 51, 55, 226–8
   rates 18–19, 107, 140, 150, 163, 166
   self care aware consulting style 41, 51, 60, 229–33
Consumer Health Information Centre (CHIC) 104, 105
contraception 65, 66, 76, 86, 97
COPD *see* chronic obstructive pulmonary disease
coronary heart disease (CHD) 7, 82, 89, 91, 96
cough
   asthma 89, 152
   evaluation 118
   minor ailment scheme 84, 86, 138
   overview of self care 5, 7
   patient pathway
      case study 159–64
      self care 165–8
   pharmacists 84, 86, 89, 138
   sore throat 131
cultural diversity 54, 56, 58, 67, 109–10

DAFNE (Dose Adjustment For Normal Eating) 21, 234
decision making 53, 59, 60–3, 108
'delayed' prescriptions 134, 168
Delivering Choosing Health 6
denial 103, 114
dentists xi, 31, 34, 46, 57, 92, 107
Department of Health (DH) 5–6, 11–12, 86, 89, 96, 234
depression 10, 20, 25, 107, 109, 142
DESMOND (Diabetes Education and Self Management for Ongoing and Newly Diagnosed) 21, 234
Developing Patient Partnerships (DPP) 21, 104, 107, 110, 234
DH *see* Department of Health
diabetes
   cough and colds 167

DESMOND 21, 234
educational interventions 19–21
long term conditions 22, 23, 87, 89
patient's perspective 104–5, 107–9
pharmacy teams 24, 82, 87, 89, 91–2, 96
promoting self care 10, 25
reliable information 58, 68
risks 75
diarrhoea 17, 84, 86, 160, 165
diet
   cough and colds 167
   educational interventions 21
   enabling patients to self care 56, 58, 59
   health and social services 9
   health inequalities 8
   patient's perspective 102, 103, 105, 109
   pharmacists 90–3
digital TV 69, 107, 234
DiPEx (Directory of Patient Experience) 94, 234
disability 61, 110, 143
DISCERN 67, 234
district nurses 32, 92, 138–9, 141, 143, 148–9
doctors *see* GPs
Dose Adjustment For Normal Eating *see* DAFNE
DPP *see* Developing Patient Partnerships
Dr Foster 104
drug misuse 9, 104

earache 18, 19, 84, 86
echinacea 167, 168
education
   asthma 157
   educational interventions 18–21
   general practice teams 46–7
   health inequalities 8, 9
   health professionals 58, 61, 69, 70
   long term conditions 22
   overview of self care 9–11, 17, 25
   patient's perspective 58, 61, 105, 108
   PCTs 35–7, 40
   personal development plans 69, 70
EHC *see* emergency hormonal contraception
elderly patients 10, 20, 99, 108
Electronic Medical Information Service (EMIS) 93

emergency care
  enabling self care 60, 66
  general practice teams 50
  PART model 17
  patient pathways 132, 150, 154, 166
  PCTs 31
  pharmacy teams 85, 86
emergency hormonal contraception (EHC) 65, 66, 86, 97
EMIS (Electronic Medical Information Service) 93
empowerment 10–12, 20–1, 60–1, 174
enhanced services 38, 81, 84, 87, 92, 95, 98
epiglottitis 132
EPP *see* Expert Patients Programme
Epstein–Barr virus (EBV) 133
Erewash PCT xii, 7, 21, 24, 98
essential services
  developing pharmacy team 94–6
  long term conditions 86–90
  minor ailment scheme 84–6
  overview 81–2
  pharmacy contract 81
  public health 90–4
  self-limiting problems 82–4
  signposting 93–4
  training needs analysis 200
ethnicity 106, 108, 109–10, 119
evaluation 36, 41, 51, 115, 118–22
exercise
  asthma 152
  back pain 136, 143, 144, 145
  cough and colds 167
  educational interventions 20
  enabling self care 56, 58, 64
  exercise on prescription 38
  health and social services 9
  health inequalities 8
  long term conditions 22, 90
  patient's perspective 102–4, 110
  pharmacy support 90–3
  sore throat 127
The Expert Patient 5
Expert Patients Programme (EPP)
  overview of self care 5, 8, 9, 19, 23
  patient's perspective 102, 106
  PCTs 31, 38
  signposting 93
  website 234
eye contact 55, 56

Family Doctor Books 105, 234
feedback
  audit 198
  change 65, 117
  consulting style 231
  education and training 36
  health professionals 55, 63, 64, 65, 108
  patient pathways 140, 150, 163
  teamwork 202
FEV_1 (forced expiratory volume in 1 second) 152
FIT magazine 104
focus groups 101, 102
force-field analysis (Tool 1) 32, 45–6, 173–5
framing risk 76
Fylde Coast Medical Services (FCMS) 86

GABHS *see* group A beta-haemolytic streptococcus
Gantt chart (Tool 7) 34, 46, 119, 191–3
gap analysis (Tool 5) 34, 38, 46, 50, 186–7
General Medical Services (GMS) contract xi, 85
general practice teams *see also* GPs; health professionals
  competence 69
  evaluation 120, 121
  long term conditions 23
  meaning of self care 4, 7
  PCTs 32, 34, 38
  risk and safety 11
  supporting self care
    stage 1: developing vision 43–9
    stage 2: choosing interventions 49–50
    stage 3: keeping going 50–1
    stage 4: monitoring and evaluation 51–2
  workload assessment xi, 206–10
general practitioners *see* GPs
glandular fever 133, 134
glucosamine 73, 74
GMS (General Medical Services) contract xi, 85
GPs (general practitioners)
  asthma 89, 122, 148–52
  back pain 136–43
  communicating risk 75
  cough and colds 159–64, 166

developing trust 57
educational interventions 18, 19
evaluation 122
general practice teams 43, 47, 48
long term conditions 23, 89
overview of self care 3–5, 7, 10–11, 14, 53
patient's perspective 107, 108
PCTs 40
pharmacy support 83, 85–6, 89–90, 93, 98
signposting 65, 66
sore throat 125–31, 134
workload assessment xi, 76, 206, 209
group A beta-haemolytic streptococcus (GABHS) 133, 134

haemoglobin A$_{1c}$ (HbA$_{1c}$) 87, 90
harm 11, 19, 68, 74, 75
Harrow PCT 92
hay fever 5, 7, 84, 85, 89
HbA$_{1c}$ *see* haemoglobin A1c
HDL (high density lipoprotein) 90
head lice 84, 86
headache 19, 84, 112
health
 educational interventions 20
 inequalities 8–9, 12, 34, 106, 119
 overview of self care 3, 4–6, 10–12
 workplace 110
Health and Safety Executive 153
health care assistants
 general practice teams 43, 48
 patient pathways 127–8, 138–9, 148–9, 151
 workload assessment xi, 76
Healthcare Commission 57, 92
health care pyramid 14
Health Development Agency 10
health education 9–11, 18–20
Health First 101
health inequalities 8–9, 12, 34, 106, 119
Health on Net 68
health professionals
 being competent 70–4
 communicating risk 74–6
 consultation content scale 223
 definition of self care 14
 enabling self care
  communication style 54–6

developing trust 56–8
 effective information 66–9
 encouraging skills 58–60
 enhancing motivation 63–5
 overview 53–4
 providing reliable information 58
 sharing decision making 60–3
 patient's perspective 108
 personal development plans 69–70
 time management 76–8
health promotion
 enabling self care 59
 health and social services 9
 long term conditions 22, 87
 overview of self care 11, 15
 PCTs 38
 pharmacy teams 84, 87, 97
 sore throat 127
HealthSpace 68
health visitors
 back pain 138–9, 141, 143
 cough and colds 160–2, 164
 PCTs 32
 smoking 92
 teamwork 49
Healthwise handbook 108
Healthy Weight Challenge 92
herbal medicine 11, 76, 101, 102, 110, 167
Heron, J 64
HGV Man 67
high density lipoprotein (HDL) 90
Hillingdon PCT 87, 99
HIV (human immunodeficiency virus) 144
holistic care 53, 55, 56, 63, 111
home remedies 11, 19, 82, 204
hospitals
 asthma 150, 152
 educational interventions 20
 enabling patients to self care 58
 long term conditions 22, 87
 PCTs 38
 sore throat 132
 support networks 24
hypertension
 educational interventions 19
 long term conditions 23
 overview of self care 10, 25
 patient's perspective 102, 109
 pharmacy teams 82, 91–4
hyperventilation 148, 152, 153

ibuprofen 73, 136, 143, 168
IMPACT programme 84
impetigo 85, 134
inequalities 8–9, 12, 34, 106, 119
inflammatory bowel disease 20
influenza 18, 19, 153, 165, 166
information
    decision making 62–3
    educational interventions 18–20
    effective use 66–9
    health professionals 53–4, 58, 62–3, 66–9
    NHS policy 6
    patient's perspective 103, 107–8
    personal development plans 69
    pharmacy teams 83, 84
    reliability 58, 107–8
    self care guides 21
    self-limiting problems 83, 84
infrastructure and resource matrix (Tool 8) 34, 38, 46, 50, 194–6
inhalers 60, 89, 146–8, 152, 154–6
international normalised ratio (INR) 23
internet
    back pain 139
    health professionals 58, 66, 68, 73, 74
    NHS Direct Online 21, 68, 94, 107, 235
    overview of self care 4, 18, 21, 24
    patient's perspective 104–7
    pharmacy teams 93
    useful resources 234–5

Joining Up Self Care xii, 21, 40, 41, 50, 157

Kaiser Permanente 22
KISS (keep it simple and short) 117
Knowledge and Skills Framework (KSF) 69

Lab Tests Online UK 234
Lambeth PCT 98, 190
language
    audit 197
    communication style 54–5
    effective information 67, 68
    health professionals 54–5, 67, 68
    overview of self care 8, 9, 23
    reliable information 107
The Lazy Exercise Guide for Busy People 104
LDL (low density lipoprotein) 90
LDPs (local delivery plans) 31, 99

leaflets
    educational interventions 18–20
    enabling self care 21, 67, 104
    lifestyle changes 90, 92, 104
    patient pathways 127–8, 138–9, 157, 162, 167
    pharmacy teams 83–4, 90, 92–4, 96–7
Learning and Employment Action Package (LEAP) 110–11
learning logs (Tool 15) 40, 50, 51, 213–14
LES (local enhanced service) 98
Lewisham PCT 190
lifestyle
    education 19, 21, 36
    enabling self care 59, 65, 68
    long term conditions 22, 90
    overview of self care 3–4, 6, 8–10, 14–15, 17
    patient's perspective 103–4, 108
    pharmacy support 82, 90–4
local delivery plans (LDPs) 31, 99
local enhanced service (LES) 98
local pharmacy committees (LPCs) 93, 99
locums 95, 96, 126
long term conditions
    general practice teams 50
    overview of self care 8, 10, 14, 15, 22–3
    patient's perspective 101, 106
    PCTs 31, 32, 38
    pharmacy teams 81–3, 86–90, 95
low density lipoprotein (LDL) 90
LPCs *see* local pharmacy committees
LungUSA 153

magnetic resonance imaging 144
Making Sense of Health xii, 108
MAS *see* minor ailment scheme
massage 73, 74, 101, 143
mastoiditis 168
medicines
    enabling self care 59, 62, 67
    patient's perspective 102
    pharmacy teams 85, 89, 90
Medicines Partnership 96, 234
medicines use review (MUR) 89, 96, 149
MEDLINEplus 234
meningitis 166
Men's Health 104
mental health
    back pain 142

Index

educational interventions 20
enabling self care 56, 59, 60
patient's perspective 101, 104, 105
pharmacy teams 86, 97
MeRec Bulletin 134
midwives 49, 68, 138, 143
MIND 104
minor ailment scheme (MAS)
    future of NHS 5
    PCTs 31, 38
    pharmacy teams 84–6, 96
    sore throat 128, 130, 135
minor ailments
    overview of self care 5, 7, 17
    patient pathways 128, 130, 135, 163
    patient's perspective 102, 104, 105, 108
    PCTs 31, 38
    pharmacy teams 81–6, 95–6
minority groups 23, 34, 106, 110
monitoring 41, 51, 89–90, 115, 117–18
motivation
    enhancing 63–5
    force-field analysis 174
    general practice teams 49
    health professionals 53, 55, 63–5
    managing change 115
    patient's perspective 101, 103, 105, 106, 109–10
moving through change (Tool 14) 40, 50, 211–12
MUR *see* medicines use review
MyPil 68

National electronic Library for Health 234
National Health Service *see* NHS
National Heart Lung and Blood Institute 148, 153
National Library for Health 234
National Patient Safety Agency (NPSA) 11
National Pharmacy Association (NPA) 96, 105
National Programme for Information Technology 68
National Service Frameworks (NSFs) 22, 188
nebulisers 24, 152
neuro-linguistic programming (NLP) 64
Newcastle-under-Lyme PCT 93
Next Moves 111
nGMS (new GMS contract) 85

NHS (National Health Service)
    back pain 73, 74
    future of NHS 4, 5–6
    overview of self care xi, 8, 10–11, 16, 25
    patient's perspective 106, 108, 112
    pharmacy teams 83, 84, 86, 92
    websites 234, 235
NHS Centre for Pharmacy Postgraduate Education 96
NHS Direct
    general practice teams 50
    overview of self care 3, 21
    patient pathways 127, 131, 139, 143, 160–1, 166
    patient's perspective 107
    pharmacy teams 83, 85, 94
NHS Direct Interactive 21, 234
NHS Direct Online 21, 68, 94, 235
NHS Improvement Plan 5
NHS Knowledge and Skills Framework (KSF) 69
The NHS Plan 5
NHS trusts 22, 104
NLP *see* neuro-linguistic programming
non-steroidal anti-inflammatory drugs (NSAIDs) 137, 138, 145, 152
non-verbal communication 56
NPA *see* National Pharmacy Association
NPSA *see* National Patient Safety Agency
NSAIDs *see* non-steroidal anti-inflammatory drugs
NSFs *see* National Service Frameworks
nurses
    asthma 122, 146–9, 151
    back pain 138–9, 141, 143
    communicating risk 75
    cough and colds 161–4
    enabling self care 53, 58–60, 65–6, 105
    evaluation 122
    general practice teams 43, 45, 48, 49
    overview of self care 3, 11, 14, 23
    pharmacy teams 83, 86, 92
    schools 32
    sore throat 126–30, 134
    workload assessment xi, 76, 206

obesity 34, 97, 105, 109, 127
older people 10, 20, 99, 108
OOH *see* out of hours care
open questions 62–3, 64, 227

orlistat (Xenical) 92
orthopaedic services 140, 141
osteoarthritis 23, 74
osteopaths 111, 143
OTC *see* over-the-counter medicines
otitis media 133, 134, 167, 168
Our Health, Our Care, Our Say 6
out of hours (OOH) care 31, 85, 86
outpatient care 10, 23, 107
over-the-counter (OTC) medicines
   communicating risk 75, 76
   complementary medicine 102
   enabling patients to self care 53, 65–6
   evaluation 121
   overview of self care 4, 5, 11
   patient pathways 128, 138
   pharmacy teams 82, 83, 85–7, 98
   significant event audit 204

P (pharmacy medicines) 65, 97
PAGB (Proprietary Association of Great Britain) 235
paracetamol 73, 125, 131, 137, 143–4, 159, 168
Parkinson's disease 19
PART model (prevention, await resolution, relief of symptoms, toleration of symptoms)
   asthma 147, 150, 153–4
   back pain 137, 140, 142–3
   components of self care 16, 17
   cough and colds 160, 163, 164, 166–7
   general practice teams 49, 50
   PCTs 38
   pharmacy teams 83
   sore throat 126, 129, 131–2
   workload assessment (Tool 13) 38, 41, 49, 50, 84, 206–10
patient group directions (PGDs) 85, 86, 92
Patient Information Publications (PiP) 93
patient medication records (PMRs) 94
patient pathways
   asthma 146–57
   back pain 136–45
   cough and colds 159–68
   general practice teams 49–50
   overview 123
   PART model 17
   sore throat 125–35

patients
   consultation content scale 223–5
   educational interventions 18, 19
   enabling self care
      communication style 54–6
      developing trust 56–8
      effective information 66–9
      enhancing motivation 63–5
      overview 53–4, 58–60
      risk 74–6
      sharing decision making 60–3
      signposting 65
   long term conditions 22–3, 87
   overview of self care 3–4, 10–12
   patient-centred care 23, 41, 47, 51, 55, 58–9, 226–8
   PCTs 31, 40
   pharmacy teams 85, 87, 96
   safety 31, 207
   satisfaction 120, 121
   shared care 14
   view of self care
      how they self care 102–5
      how to improve 105–12
      overview 101–2
Patient UK 68, 93
Patient Voices 235
PCTs *see* primary care trusts
PDSA (plan, do, study, act) (Tool 6) 34, 46, 188–90
penicillin 134
performance 70, 118, 202
personal development plans 47, 69–70, 217, 218
personal support mapping (Tool 18) 41, 51, 78, 221–2
PEST (political, economic, sociological and technological) (Tool 4) 34, 46, 183–5
Pfizer Health Solutions 22
PGDs *see* patient group directions
Pharmaceutical Services Negotiating Committee (PSNC) 95
pharmacists
   asthma 122, 147–8, 149, 151
   back pain 138, 141
   contract 31, 81, 84, 93, 96–9, 108
   cough and colds 160–4, 168
   evaluation 120–2
   general practice teams 43, 45, 46, 49

Index

overview of self care 4–5, 7–8, 10, 14, 17, 21
patient's perspective 107, 108
PCTs 31, 32, 34, 36, 38
sore throat 125, 127–31
supporting self care
    developing team 94–6, 99–100
    long term conditions 86–90
    minor ailment scheme 84–6
    overview 53, 81–2, 99–100
    pharmacy contract 81
    public health 90–4
    quality and audit 97–8
    self-limiting problems 82–4
    signposting 66, 93–4
teamwork 24, 81, 95–6, 99–100, 108
workload xi
Pharmacy Alliance 87, 89
Pharmacy First 7, 24
pharmacy medicines (P) 65, 97
physiotherapy 43, 49, 104, 138–41, 143, 148–9
Pilgrim Projects 235
PiP (Patient Information Publications) 93
placebo effect 112
Plain English Campaign 68
plan, do, study, act *see* PDSA
PLIs *see* prescription-linked interventions
PMRs (patient medication records) 94
pneumonia 166, 167
POM *see* prescription only medicines
portfolios 69–70, 72, 74, 213
PR *see* public relations
practice managers
    general practice teams 43, 48
    patient pathways 127–8, 138–41, 148–9, 151, 161–2, 164
practice nurses
    asthma 148, 149, 151
    back pain 138
    cough and colds 161, 164
    enabling self care 58, 59–60
    general practice teams 48
    overview of self care 14
    sore throat 126–7, 129–30
prednisolone 152, 156
prescription-linked interventions (PLIs) 91–3, 95, 96
prescription only medicines (POM) 65, 83, 85, 92, 97–8

prescriptions
    NHS policy 5
    patient pathways 127, 128, 134, 138, 148, 167
    pharmacy teams 83–6, 91–3, 95–8
    significant event audit 204
    signposting 65–6
primary care
    general practice teams 43
    health professionals 53, 54, 57
    overview of self care vii, xi, 4, 7–8, 25
    pharmacy teams 81, 98–9
primary care trusts (PCTs)
    competence 69
    evaluation 41, 118–21
    general practice teams 43
    long term conditions 22
    overview of self care vii, 4, 7–8, 11
    patient pathways 128, 130, 139, 149, 151, 162, 164
    patient's perspective 104, 106
    pharmacy teams 84–6, 90, 92–3, 96–9
    supporting self care
        action plan 34
        building teamwork 38
        choosing interventions 38
        education and training 35–7
        keeping going 39–41
        monitoring and evaluation 41
        overview 30–4, 39
        priorities and target groups 35
        resource mapping 34–5
    WiPP xi, xii
priorities 35, 38, 41, 46, 49–52, 76, 179–80
priority checklist (Tool 17) 41, 51, 69, 95, 217–20
Prodigy 21, 127, 144, 162
Proprietary Association of Great Britain (PAGB) 235
protocols 94, 121, 122, 130
PSNC (Pharmaceutical Services Negotiating Committee) 95
public health 36, 38, 82, 84, 86, 90–5
public relations (PR) 8, 32

quality 69, 96, 197–9
Quality and Outcomes Framework (QOF) 7, 31, 90, 188
quinsy 17, 132, 134

rapport 54, 55, 57, 63
re-framing 64, 103
reception staff
  general practice teams 43, 48
  patient pathways 126–30, 138–9, 141, 148–9, 151, 161, 164
  training 36
record keeping 82–3, 91, 93, 94, 96
'red flags' 17, 132, 144
reduce time pressures (Tool 16) 40, 51, 215–16
referrals 17, 25, 82–3, 85, 93–4, 141
religion 103, 110, 119, 122
repeat prescriptions 99, 148
resource mapping 34–5, 46 *see also* infrastructure and resource matrix
rheumatic fever 133, 134
rhinitis 133, 157, 165
risk
  communicating 74–6
  educational interventions 21
  effective information 68
  overview of self care 8, 11, 14, 19, 25
  PCTs 31
Royal College of Physicians 89
Royal National Institute of the Blind (RNIB) 68
Royal Pharmaceutical Society of Great Britain (RPSGB) 97, 105
Rugby PCT 93

safety 11, 31, 69, 83, 120–2, 207
salbutamol 152
scarlet fever 133, 134
schools xii, 9, 32, 92, 134, 143, 165
sciatica 142
Scottish Intercollegiate Guidelines Network (SIGN) 127, 134, 148, 157
secondary care 25, 31, 140, 144, 150
Securing our Future Health 5
self-assessment 18, 21, 217, 218–20
Self Care – a real choice 6
self care
  definitions vii, 14, 102
  evaluation 118–22
  managing change 114–17
  practice and impact
    affordability 25
    assistive technologies 24
    components 16–18

    educational interventions 18–21
    long term conditions 22–3
    overview 14–16
    support networks 24
  supporting
    general practice teams 4, 7
    health inequalities 8–9
    integrated strategy 7–8
    from medical to self care 10
    NHS policy 4–6
    overview 11–12
    promoting health and wellbeing 10–11
    public view of 3
    risk and safety 11
  useful resources 234
  WiPP xii
self care aware consulting style (Tool 21) 41, 51, 60, 229–33
Self Care for People xii, 60
Self Care for Primary Healthcare Professionals xii
self help 20, 24, 25, 68, 108
self-limiting problems 81–6, 95, 102 *see also* minor ailments
self-monitoring 10, 15, 23, 25, 38, 58, 105
sexual health 66, 104, 105
shared care 9, 14
shared decision making 60–3
sickness absence 21, 110, 142
side-effects 57, 59, 66, 76, 102, 111, 134
SIGN *see* Scottish Intercollegiate Guidelines Network
significant event audit (Tool 12) 38, 40–1, 47, 50–1, 204–5
signposting 53, 65–6, 82, 91, 93–5, 120–1, 197
simvastatin 97, 98
sinusitis 133, 134, 167, 168
smoking
  asthma 153, 154
  cough and colds 167, 168
  enabling self care 65, 68
  health and social services 9
  health inequalities 8
  PART model 16, 38
  patient's perspective 104, 108
  pharmacy support 82, 91–2, 96, 97
  risk 75
  sore throat 127, 131
social inclusion partnerships (SIPs) 91

Index

social services 9, 11, 31, 38, 86
SOPs *see* standard operating procedures
sore throat
   complementary medicine 102
   cough and colds 165, 166
   educational interventions 19
   evaluation 118
   PART model 17
   patient pathway
      case study 125–30
      self care 131–5
   pharmacy support 84, 86
Southwark PCT 98, 190
spacers 146, 152
spondylitis 142, 144
St John's wort 76
standard operating procedures (SOPs) 94, 95
StaRNeT website assessment tool (SWAT) 68
steroids 152, 154, 156
Stop Smoking services 91–2, 104
strategy 30–2, 39, 43, 46, 118–20
strategy and action plan (Tool 2) 32, 36, 46, 176–80
stress 59, 77–8, 91, 142
sunburn 104, 133
support networks
   enabling self care 54, 58–9, 66–8
   overview of self care 3, 9, 22, 24
   patient's perspective 104, 108
   personal support mapping (Tool 18) 41, 51, 78, 221–2
   time management 77, 78
Supporting People with Long Term Conditions to Self Care 6
Sure Start 17, 24
SWAT (StaRNeT website assessment tool) 68
SWOT analysis (strengths, weaknesses, opportunities, threats) (Tool 3) 32, 35, 38, 46, 50, 181–2

Tate, P 223
Taunton Deane PCT 85
team function checklist (Tool 11) 38, 40, 47, 51, 202–3
teamwork
   asthma 147–8, 151
   back pain 137, 141

   cough and colds 160–1, 164
   evaluation 119, 121
   general practice 45, 47–9, 51
   PCTs 38, 40
   pharmacists 24, 95, 97
   sore throat 126, 130
   training needs analysis 200–1
   workload assessment 206–10
thrush 85
time management 40, 51, 76–8, 215–16
timetabling 34, 46, 191–3
Tools overview 33, 44, 171
Tool 1: force-field analysis 32, 45–6, 173–5
Tool 2: strategy and action plan 32, 36, 46, 176–80
Tool 3: SWOT analysis 32, 35, 38, 46, 50, 181–2
Tool 4: PEST 34, 46, 183–5
Tool 5: gap analysis 34, 38, 46, 50, 186–7
Tool 6: PDSA 34, 46, 188–90
Tool 7: Gantt chart 34, 46, 119, 191–3
Tool 8: infrastructure and resource matrix 34, 38, 46, 50, 194–6
Tool 9: audit 35, 41, 46, 51, 197–9
Tool 10: training needs analysis 36, 40, 46–7, 51, 69, 95, 200–1
Tool 11: team function checklist 38, 40, 47, 51, 202–3
Tool 12: significant event audit 38, 40–1, 47, 50–1, 204–5
Tool 13: PART/workload assessment 38, 41, 49, 50, 84, 206–10
Tool 14: moving through change 40, 50, 211–12
Tool 15: learning log 40, 50, 51, 213–14
Tool 16: reduce time pressures 40, 51, 215–16
Tool 17: priority checklist 41, 51, 69, 95, 217–20
Tool 18: personal support mapping 41, 51, 78, 221–2
Tool 19: consultation content scale 41, 51, 55, 223–5
Tool 20: consulting style scale 41, 51, 55, 226–8
Tool 21: self care aware consulting style 41, 51, 60, 229–33
Towards a DH/NHS Strategy to Support Self Care 5

training
  audit 197, 198
  evaluation 119–21
  general practice teams 43, 45, 46–7
  health professionals 54, 60, 65, 69
  overview of self care 3, 5–9, 11
  PCTs 30–1, 32, 35–7, 40, 41
  pharmacy teams 94, 96, 98
  WiPP xi, xii
training needs analysis (Tool 10) 36, 40, 46–7, 51, 69, 95, 200–1
triage 11, 83, 86, 162, 206
trust 9, 53, 56–8, 101, 108
TV services 69, 107, 234

ulcerative colitis 21, 23
unconscious (in)competence 72
unemployment 61, 110–11
'Up for it?' programme 91
upper respiratory tract infection (URTI) 152, 157, 166
urinary tract infection 85

videos 18, 138, 225, 229, 231
viruses 133, 165, 167
vitamin C 167, 168
voluntary groups 3, 20, 31, 34, 46, 106

walk-in centres (WICs) 83, 86

Walsall PCT 84
Wanless, D 5, 10, 25, 30
warfarin 23, 76
websites 68, 73–4, 93, 107, 139, 234–5
  see also internet
weight management 64, 67, 90–3, 99, 108
wellbeing 3, 5–6, 9–12, 20, 56, 110
WICs *see* walk-in centres
work 8, 66, 110–11, 134, 142–3, 153
Working in Partnership Programme (WiPP)
  general practice teams 43, 45, 50
  overview xi, 123
  patient's perspective 108
  PCTs 30
  pharmacy teams 93
  website 235
workload
  assessment (Tool 13) 38, 41, 49, 50, 84, 206–10
  force-field analysis 174
  time management xi, 40, 51, 76–8, 215–16
workshops 49, 51, 96, 99

Xenical (orlistat) 92

yellow flags 142